Landmark Papers in Neurosurgery

Edited by

Reuben D. Johnson, DPhil, FRCS (Neuro.Surg)

Alexander L. Green, MD, FRCS (SN)

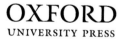

OXFORD
UNIVERSITY PRESS

OXFORD

UNIVERSITY PRESS

Great Clarendon Street, Oxford ox2 6DP

Oxford University Press is a department of the University of Oxford.
It furthers the University's objective of excellence in research, scholarship,
and education by publishing worldwide in

Oxford New York

Auckland Cape Town Dar es Salaam Hong Kong Karachi
Kuala Lumpur Madrid Melbourne Mexico City Nairobi
New Delhi Shanghai Taipei Toronto

With offices in

Argentina Austria Brazil Chile Czech Republic France Greece Guatemala
Hungary Italy Japan Poland Portugal Singapore South
Korea Switzerland Thailand Turkey Ukraine Vietnam

Oxford is a registered trade mark of Oxford University Press
in the UK and in certain other countries

Published in the United States
by Oxford University Press Inc., New York

British Library Cataloguing in Publication Data
Data available

Library of Congress Cataloging in Publication Data
Data available

Typeset in Minion by Glyph International, Bangalore, India
Printed in Great Britain
on acid-free paper by
The MPG Books Group, Bodmin and King's Lynn

ISBN 978–0–19–959125–1

10 9 8 7 6 5 4 3 2 1

Foreword

Joseph C. Maroon

While reviewing this volume on *Landmark Papers in Neurosurgery*, I thought of another book presented to me at the completion of my training at the Radcliffe Infirmary in Oxford—too many years ago. Mr Brian Cummins, then Senior Registrar, regularly thrashed me on the squash courts (although not *that* skilled!) next to the Radcliffe, when not on call. He shared his winning secret with the presentation of the classic—*The Theory and Practice of Gamesmanship or The Art of Winning Games without Actually Cheating* by Stephen Potter, another Oxonian. This volume by Reuben Johnson and Alexander Green is the ultimate neurosurgical 'gamesmanship' book for whoever reads it. For the resident, seminal large complex investigative studies—'game changing' themselves—are analysed, summarized, and then superbly critiqued. The essence of major papers such as the optimal timing for aneurysm surgery, the use of nimodipine, and the indications for decompressive surgery for the management of malignant cerebral infarction can be easily 'dropped' on rounds or in conferences with the appearance of having spent hours doing the same meticulous analysis as the authors—without really cheating! For the neurosurgical/neurological faculty, a few quick minutes are all it takes to refresh one's own database and present a learned discussion or lecture on the history of the use of steroids for cerebral oedema, the rationale for the extent of resection for malignant gliomas, the use of barbiturates in head injury or how magnesium is neuroprotective in brain injuries.

For all in the neurosciences, the authors have distilled thousands of hours of literature review into concise, easily read, and critiqued summaries of papers on head injury, the treatment of spine and spinal cord diseases and functional neurosurgery that are delightful to read and immediately practical in everyday patient care. Having participated in journal clubs and literature reviews for 25 years, this book, a landmark itself, has the obviousness of so many great innovations that makes the person reading it ask the question—why didn't I think of this myself? The scientific base and perspective gained from such a critical review of past neurosurgical classics prods the reader to look into the future of our specialty and ask, what's next? In his letter to Robert Hook on 5 February 1675 Isaac Newton wrote, 'If I have seen farther, it is by standing on the shoulders of giants'.

With these landmark studies the authors have hoisted us high onto the shoulders of neurosurgical giants and the view of the past (as herein beautifully presented), the present, and the future of neurosurgery is breathtaking.

Joseph C. Maroon
Professor and Heindl Scholar in Neuroscience
Department of Neurological Surgery
University of Pittsburgh School of Medicine;

Team Neurosurgeon, Pittsburgh Steelers
Pittsburgh, Pennsylvania, USA

Landmark Papers in Neurosurgery

Landmark Papers in... series

Titles in the series

Landmark Papers in Neurosurgery
Edited by Reuben D. Johnson and Alexander L. Green

Landmark Papers in Anaesthesia
Edited by Nigel Webster and Helen Galley

Landmark Papers in Cardiology
Edited by Aung Myat and Tony Gershlick

Foreword

Angelo Franzini

Neurosurgery is a lover who becomes ever younger while we grow older. Reading this book, I fell in love again with this young lady. I appreciated the enthusiasm of the authors who have solid experience in the field in reporting new perspectives and leading the reader through the chapters. Clear and understandable guidelines for each of the topics addressed in this book are presented for approaching the problems under discussion. The lectures demonstrate that it takes much longer to understand the indications for a specific surgical procedure than to learn how to perform the hands-on surgical procedure itself.

Moreover, the authors remind us that the management of CNS diseases in many instances may be controversial. The choice between more conservative and more aggressive 'radical' treatments may be difficult as in the surgical treatment of trigeminal neuralgia or even that of intracranial aneurysms. Reports from up-to-date cooperative studies in the chapter dedicated to neurovascular diseases make this book particularly rich and realistic at the same time.

A full range of theories and approaches are clearly examined to 'educate' both young and old neurosurgeons. Many of them too often focus their attention on a narrow sub-speciality topic such as cranial base surgery, functional neurosurgery, or spinal surgery.

A complete knowledge of all the fields of interest in neurosurgery is clearly not possible, but this book reminds us that many concepts are common and many surgical techniques must be shared among different neurosurgical applications. Endoscopy, neuronavigation, microsurgery, and stereotaxis are common instruments that all neurosurgeons must know in order to offer their patients the best therapeutic options.

Travelling through this book, neurosurgeons become aware of the fact that the knowledge of many other disciplines is mandatory in accomplishing that task. Anatomy and physiology are not enough. We need to know functional neuroimaging, physics, genetics, statistics, informatics, and computer technology … read this book.

Angelo Franzini
Neurosurgeon in Milan

Contents

Contributors

Arnar Astradsson
Copenhagen University Clinic of
Neurosurgery
Copenhagen
Denmark

Tipu Z. Aziz
Department of Neurosurgery
John Radcliffe Hospital
Oxford
UK

Mark Bernstein
Department of Neurosurgery
Toronto Western Hospital
Toronto
Ontario
Canada

Simon A. Cudlip
Department of Neurosurgery
John Radcliffe Hospital
Oxford
UK

Katherine J. Drummond
Department of Neurosurgery
University of Melbourne
Parkville
Victoria
Australia

Alexander L. Green
Department of Neurosurgery
John Radcliffe Hospital
Oxford
UK

Jay Jayamohan
Department of Neurosurgery
John Radcliffe Hospital
Headley Way
Oxford
UK

Reuben D. Johnson
Department of Neurosurgery
John Radcliffe Hospital
Oxford
UK
Department of Neurosurgery
Royal Melbourne Hospital
Parkville
Victoria
Australia

Richard S. C. Kerr
Department of Neurosurgery
John Radcliffe Hospital
Oxford
UK

Kathleen J. O. L. Khu
Department of Neurosurgery
Toronto Western Hospital
Toronto
Ontario
Canada

John C. D. Leach
Department of Neurosurgery
Hope Hospital
Salford
Manchester
UK

Willem Adriaan Liebenberg
Paarl Medi Clinic
Paarl
Western Province
South Africa

Nicholas Maartens
Department of Neurosurgery
Royal Melbourne Hospital
Parkville
Victoria
Australia

Peter Richards
Department of Neurosurgery
John Radcliffe Hospital
Headley Way
Oxford
UK

Thomas Santarius
Department of Neurosurgery
Addenbrooke's Hospital
Cambridge
UK

Saurabh Sinha
Sheffield Children's Hospital
Sheffield
South Yorkshire
UK

Richard J. Stacey
Department of Neurosurgery
John Radcliffe Hospital
Oxford
UK

Jack E. Wilberger
Department of Neurosurgery
Allegheny General Hospital
Drexel University School of Medicine
Pittsburgh
Pennsylvania
USA

Abbreviations

5-ALA	5-aminolevulinic acid	CT	Computed tomography
A.comm	Anterior communicating artery	CTA	Computerized tomography angiography
ACA	Anterior cerebral artery	CVP	Central venous pressure
ACAS	Asymptomatic Carotid Atherosclerosis Study	DBI	Diffuse brain injury
ALT	Alanine aminotransferase	DBS	Deep brain stimulation
APACHE	Acute Physiology and Chronic Health Evaluation	DECIMAL	Decompressive craniectomy in malignant MCA infarction
ARR	Absolute risk reduction	DECRA	DECompressive CRANiectomy Trial
ASCI	Acute spinal cord injury	DESTINY	Decompressive surgery for the treatment of malignant infarction of the MCA
ASDH	Acute subdural haematoma		
ASIA	American Spinal Injury Association		
AVM	Arteriovenous malformation	DID	Delayed ischaemic deficit
BCNU	1,3-bis (2-chloroethyl)-1-nitrosourea or carmustine	DIND	Delayed ischaemic neurological deficit
BCT	Best conventional therapy	DSM-IV	Diagnostic and Statistical Manual of Mental Disorders, 4th edition
BFMDRS	Burke–Fahn–Marsden Dystonia Rating Scale		
CA	Carcinoma	DXT	Deep X-ray therapy
CAVATAS	Carotid And Vertebral Artery Transluminal Angioplasty Study	EBRT	External beam radiation therapy
		ECOG	Eastern Cooperative Oncology Group
CDM	Conventional dose mannitol		
CES	Cauda equina syndrome	ECST	European Carotid Surgery Trial
Cg25	Cingulate gyrus area 25	ECT	Electroconvulsive therapy
Cg25WM	Subgenual cingulate white matter	EDH	Extradural haematoma
		EEG	Electroencephalogram
CLEAR IVH	Clot Lysis: Evaluating Accelerated Resolution of Intraventricular Hemorrhage	EORTC	European Organisation for Research and Treatment of Cancer Brain Tumour and Radiotherapy Group
CMM	Conventional medical management	EVA-3S	Endarterectomy Versus Angioplasty in Patients with Symptomatic Severe Carotid Stenosis trial
CNS	Central nervous system		
CPP	Cerebral perfusion pressure		
CRASH	Corticosteroids Randomization After Significant Head injury trial	EVD	Extraventricular drain
		FBSS	Failed back surgery syndrome
		FIS	Functional Independent Survival
CREST	Carotid Revascularization Endarterectomy versus Stenting Trial	GBM	Glioblastoma multiforme
		GCS	Glasgow Coma Scale
CSDH	Chronic subdural haematoma	GI	Gastrointestinal
CSF	Cerebrospinal fluid	GM	Grey matter

GOS	Glasgow Outcome Scale	MRC	Medical Research Council
GOSE	Glasgow Outcome Scale Extended	MRI	Magnetic resonance imaging
		mRS	Modified Rankin score
GPi	Globus pallidus internus	MVD	Microvascular decompression
GSG	Gliadel Study Group	NASCET	North American Symptomatic Carotid Endarterectomy Trial
HAMLET	Hemicraniectomy after MAC infarction with life threatening oedema trial	NASCIS	National Acute Spinal Cord Injury Study
HDM	High dose mannitol	NCCTG	North Center Cancer Treatment Group
HDRS	Hamilton Depression Rating Scale	NCIC CTG	National Cancer Institute of Canada Clinical Trials Group
HeADDFIRST	Hemicraniectomy and durotomy on deterioration from infarction-related swelling trial	NHS	National Health Service
		NSAIDs	Non-steroidal anti-inflammatory drugs
HHH	Hypertension, hypervolaemia, and haemodilution	NYIAVMS	New York Islands AVM Study
HSS	Hypertonic saline solution	OCD	Obsessive compulsive disorder
HSU	Health State Utility	ODI	Oswestry Disability Index
ICA	Internal carotid artery	P.comm	Posterior communicating artery
ICH	Intracerebral haemorrhage	PAWP	Pulmonary artery wedge pressure
ICP	Intracranial pressure		
ICSS	International Carotid Stenting Study	PBTTG	Polymer Brain Tumour Treatment Group
IPH	Intraparenchymal haematoma	PCA	Posterior cerebral artery
ISAT	International Subarachnoid Aneurysm trial	PCPC	Paediatric cerebral performance category scale
ISUIA	International Study of Unruptured Intracranial Aneurysms	PD	Parkinson's disease
		PDQ-39	Parkinson's Disease Questionaire
		PET	Positron emission tomography
IV	Intravenous	PFS	Progression-free survival
IVH	Intraventricular haemorrhage	PHVD	Post-haemorrhagic ventricular dilatation
JROSG	Japanese Radiation Oncology Study Group		
		PO	Per os
KPS	Karnofsky Performance Score	PRCT	Placebo-controlled randomized trial
LP	Lumbar puncture		
MCA	Middle cerebral artery	PROCESS	Prospective Randomized Controlled Multi-centre Trial of the Effectiveness of Spinal Cord Stimulation
MePred	Methyl prednisolone		
MESCC	Metastatic spinal cord compression		
		PTS	Post-traumatic seizures
MGMT	O^6-methylguanine DNA methyltransferase	QOL	Quality of life
		QOLIE	Quality of life inventory (Epilepsy)
MISTIE	Minimally Invasive Surgery plus rt-PA for Intracerebral Hemorrhage Evaluation		
		RCT	Randomized controlled trial
mJOA	Modified Japanese Association Scale	RESCUE-ICP	Randomized Evaluation of Surgery with Craniectomy for Uncontollable Elevation of Intra-Cranial Pressure
MMI	Malignant MCA infarction		

REZ	Root entry zone		STICH	International Surgical Trial in Intracerebral Haemorrhage
RPA	Recursive partitioning analysis		STIMEP	Assessment of Subthalamic Nucleus Stimulation in Drug Resistant Epilepsy
RR	Relative risk			
RTOG	Radiation Therapy Oncology Group		STN	Subthalamic nucleus
SAH	Subarachnoid haemorrhage		SWT	Shuttle-walking test
SANTE	Stimulation of the Anterior Nucleus of the Thalamus in Epilepsy		TBI	Traumatic brain injury
			TCD	Transcranial Doppler
			TH	Tyrosine hydroxylase
SAPPHIRE	Stenting and Angioplasty with Protection in Patients of High Risk for Endarterectomy		THAM	Tromomethamine
			TIA	Transient ischaemic attack
SBI	Sciatica Botherness Index		TN	Trigeminal neuralgia
SCS	Spinal cord stimulation		TRISS	Trauma and Injury Severity Score
SDH	Subdural haematoma			
SF-36	Medical Outcomes Study 36-Item Short Form General Health Survey		TTP	Time to progression
			UPDRS	Unified Parkinson's Disease Rating Scale
SIVMS	Scottish Intracranial Vascular Malformation Study		VAS	Visual analogue scale
SPACE	Stent-Protected Angioplasty versus Carotid Endarterectomy study		VM	Ventral midbrain
			VNS	Vagal nerve stimulation
			WBRT	Whole brain radiotherapy
SPORT	Spine Patient Outcomes Research Trial		WFNS	World Federation of Neurological Surgeons
SRS	Stereotactic radiosurgery		WM	White matter
SSRIs	Selective serotonin reuptake inhibitors			
STASH	SimvaSTatin in Aneurysmal Subarachnoid Haemorrhage			

Introduction

The absence of proof does not constitute the proof of absence.

Virchow (1880)

The correct treatment of a potentially lethal lesion depends upon an accurate knowledge of its natural history.

Wylie McKissock (1965)

What constitutes a landmark paper in neurosurgery is highly subjective. In a field as extensive as neurosurgery how can one really pick out a group of studies and say that they are more important than all the others? Any study that has significantly changed the neurosurgical specialty is certainly a landmark study and this will include those studies that have led to a paradigm shift in accepted methods of treating neurosurgical pathology. Studies that affect management decisions for common neurosurgical conditions are also landmark studies. This includes not only clinical trials of treatment modalities but also large epidemiological studies that elucidate the natural history of a disorder. In this volume, we have attempted to include those studies that we feel primarily fall into these two groups. As a result the neurovascular, neuro-oncology and head injury chapters form the larger chapters. In addition, we have included studies that have made a significant attempt to answer an important neurosurgical question even if they have not yet provided a satisfactory answer. In our view at least, these studies should be classified as landmarks, as they will highlight the difficulties of trying to design and carry out such studies in neurosurgical patients. However, in this volume we have not endeavoured to produce a 'role of honour' of classic studies in neurosurgery, although many such studies have been referenced in the introduction to chapters and in the critiques of individual studies. In this way, there will, at the very least, be a doffing of our caps to such classic studies even if they have not been overtly included in this volume. Furthermore, although this volume is a collection of critiques of landmark studies rather than an evidence-based review of neurosurgery *per se*, we feel it is useful, where appropriate to stratify studies into the evidence class they represent. There are numerous methods to stratify clinical evidence and in this volume we have adopted the three-tier classification of evidence for therapeutic effectiveness based on that endorsed by the American Association of Neurological Surgeons and the Congress of Neurological Surgeons. This consists of three tiers as follows:

Class I	Well-designed, randomized, controlled trial
Class II	Well-designed comparative clinical study, e.g. non-randomized cohort study or a case-control study
Class III	Case series, comparative study with historical controls, or case reports

This classification system gives an assessment of the degree of certainty regarding the results of a study. The certainty is proportionate to the class of study with Class I, II, and III reflecting high, moderate, and unclear certainties respectively. It should be noted that we are applying this scheme to individual studies in order to make our assessment as to what class of evidence the study represents. We would also emphasize that the classification of each study is based on our own assessment. We would, for example, classify a randomized trial that did not include a power calculation as a Class II study rather than a Class I study.

There are some studies that, although arguably landmark studies in the field of neurosurgery, have been omitted, which will need some brief explanation. We have avoided, for example, as much as possible case series that describe important advances in surgical technique. The reason for this is because it is specifically not our aim to chart the development of surgical techniques. In addition, we feel that surgical technique is also a matter of apprenticeship and schooling. The surgical methods a surgeon uses will be a product of his or her individual training and those aspects of their masters' craft they found most effective in their hands. This is part of the surgical art that is still a matter for the individual, and rightly so. The diversity in neurosurgical techniques is part of the rich tapestry of our specialty. However, we have included case series that have influenced neurosurgical practice. A case series may illustrate an important issue about the timing of surgery or provide valuable information about long-term outcomes following surgical intervention.

This volume is intended to be an informative tool to neurosurgical trainees and a useful review for practising senior neurosurgeons. Our overall aims are two-fold. Firstly, to provide a succinct review and critique of the published studies. In many ways, this volume could be said to represent a minimum *corpus sapiendi* of the larger and more influential studies in neurosurgery. This we hope will act as an introduction to the literature to trainees and in particular those coming up to exams. We have, therefore, included below a brief discussion on the issues of trial design and also a brief explanation of some of the more common terms used in clinical trials. We also hope that this volume may be of interest to established neurosurgeons who have lived through the development of our specialty into what it is today.

We have primarily focused on the main results of studies that we feel are the most important and relevant. This usually equates to the primary outcome data in most studies. However, we have included secondary outcomes where these address key questions or dilemmas that need to be highlighted for completion. Similarly, we have been fairly unforgiving of post-hoc analyses, but have endeavoured to include these where they provide important insights or may form the basis for further studies or trial designs. In this way, we may be criticized for giving an incomplete view of the findings of some studies. This is not our intention, but rather to highlight the take-home messages of the study so that they can be more easily remembered by the reader. In addition, we would emphasize that these critiques are our own interpretation of the studies and a review of published criticisms and we hope that these prove a valuable starting point for further reading.

Reuben D. Johnson & Alexander L. Green
Oxford, 2010

Chapter 1

Neurovascular neurosurgery

AL Green, RD Johnson, RSC Kerr

1.0 **Introduction**

The demonstration of a low mortality-rate by a new technique is of no value until an acceptable statistical method of assessment of the natural prognosis and of the proposed treatment is available.

Wylie McKissock (1965)

The first clinical trial performed in the field of neurovascular surgery was carried out by Wylie McKissock, Alan Richardson, and Lawrence Walsh at Atkinson Morley's Hospital, St George's, in London between 1958 and 1965, when they compared conservative and surgical treatment of anterior communicating aneurysms (McKissock *et al.*, 1965). The results of the trial did not show any difference in mortality between the two groups. The surgical methods used varied throughout the trial to include aneurysmal clipping, ligation of the proximal anterior cerebral artery, wrapping the aneurysm with muslin, and ligation of the common carotid artery. Although the results did not show any benefit from surgical intervention, this single-centre study stands out as a landmark in neurosurgery for several reasons. Firstly, it is the first attempt at a randomized controlled trial (RCT) of surgical management of a common neurosurgical disorder. Secondly, the author's rationale for carrying out the trial was not just to evaluate surgery but to further elucidate the natural history of the lesion being treated. This point is of particular importance when considering current dilemmas that face the neurosurgeon, such as the management of unruptured intracranial aneurysms and spontaneous non-aneurysmal haematomas. Thirdly, the authors emphasize the limitations of carrying out single-centre studies in neurosurgery and indicate the need for large multi-centre studies.

We have been highly selective in the studies included in this chapter and have included those studies that we feel remain true to the founding principles of the McKissock trial. The first sections of this chapter deal with aneurysmal subarachnoid haemorrhage and we have included studies that examine the natural history of aneurysms and their treatment. We have included, therefore, the International Cooperative Study by Kassell, which addresses the timing of aneurysm surgery and prognostic factors associated with good and poor outcomes. We have also included the large study of unruptured aneurysms by the International Study of Unruptured Intracranial Aneurysms Investigators (ISUIA), which is an ongoing study addressing one of the most important and controversial problems facing neurovascular surgeons. The International Subarachnoid Aneurysm Trial (ISAT) has been included because of the widespread and profound influence this study has exerted on the management of ruptured intracranial aneurysms. As vasospasm is the greatest cause of neurological morbidity in patients who survive their primary aneurysmal bleed we have also included studies of strategies for the prevention and treatment of vasospasm associated with aneurysmal subarachnoid haemorrhage. We have included strategies for which there is an accepted evidence base, such as nimodipine, and which have become accepted practice, such as 'HHH' (hypertension, hypervolaemia, and haemodilution) therapy. In addition, we have included some studies that evaluate strategies that have been promising and for which the results of ongoing trials are keenly awaited, e.g. the use of statins. In a subsequent section of the chapter, the treatment of arteriovenous malformations (AVMs) is considered. The decision to treat AVMs depends on balancing the risk of treatment versus the natural history of AVMs. Unfortunately, the natural history of AVMs has been extremely difficult to elucidate, although there are two ongoing population-based studies in Scotland and New York. Nonetheless, the Spetzler–Martin grading system is a landmark in neurosurgery as it has produced an objective system by which outcome and risks of treatment can be applied to individuals with AVMs and for this reason it has been considered (Spetzler and Martin, 1986; Hamilton and Spetzler, 1994). Further sections of this chapter deal with the surgical management of spontaneous non-aneurysmal intraparenchymal haemorrhages (STICH trial) and decompressive surgery for the management of malignant MCA infarction (DESTINY, DECIMAL, HAMLET, and HeaDFIRST trials). The final sections deal with the role of surgery in the management of carotid artery stenosis (NASCET and SPACE trials). There are, of course, some studies that many would consider to be conspicuous by their absence in this chapter. For example, there are some early classic studies demonstrating angiographic vasospasm, evaluating prognostic factors in subarachnoid haemorrhage, and determining the clinical manifestations and time course of vasospasm (Ecker and Riemenschneider, 1951; Stornelli and French, 1963; Fisher et al., 1977; Weir et al., 1978). There are numerous other examples that could have been included. However, we have endeavoured to keep each chapter concise and to include a selection of the largest published studies that cover most of the areas of neurovascular surgery that are relevant to the every day practice of all neurosurgeons. We envisage that in future editions of this volume we will be able to include a critique of large studies on endovascular techniques (angioplasty and pharmacological techniques) to treat vasospasm.

Ecker A, Riemenschneider PA. Arteriographic demonstration of spasm of the intracranial arteries, with reference to saccular arterial aneurysms. *J Neurosurg* 1951; **8**: 660–667.

Fisher CM, Roberson GH, Ojemann RG. Cerebral vasospasm with ruptured saccular aneurysm – the clinical manifestations. *Neurosurgery* 1977; **1**: 245–248.

McKissock W, Richardson A, Walsh L. Anterior communicating aneurysms: a trial of conservative and surgical treatment. *Lancet* 1965; **1**: 873–876.

Stornelli SA, French JD. Subarachnoid hemorrhage factors in prognosis and management. *J Neurosurg* 1964; **21**: 769–780.

Weir B. Grace M, Hansen J, Rothberg C. Time course of vasospasm in man. *J Neurosurg* 1978; **48**: 173–178.

1.1 **Timing of aneurysm surgery**

Details of study

The International Cooperative Study on the Timing of Aneurysm Surgery Study was the first large-scale study to look at this issue. Between December 1980 and July 1983 a total of 3521 patients were recruited out of 8879 patients with subarachnoid haemorrhage (SAH). In addition to looking at the timing aspect of surgery, many other factors that influence outcome were addressed.

Study references

Main references

There are two main references for the study: part 1 (overall management results) and part 2 (surgical results). Both are reviewed here.

Kassell NF, Torner JC, Haley EC Jr, Jane JA, Adams HP, Kongable GL. The International Cooperative Study on the Timing of Aneurysm Surgery. Part 1: overall management results. *J Neurosurg* 1990; **73**: 18–36.

Kassell NF, Torner JC, Jane JA, Haley EC Jr, Adams HP. The International Cooperative Study on the Timing of Aneurysm Surgery. Part 2: surgical results. *J Neurosurg* 1990; **73**: 37–47.

Related references

Graff-Radford NR, Torner J, Adams HP Jr, Kassell NF. Factors associated with hydrocephalus after subarachnoid hemorrhage. A report of the Cooperative Aneurysm Study. *Arch Neurol* 1989; **46**: 744–752.

Kassell NF, Torner JC. The International Cooperative Study on Timing of Aneurysm Surgery – an update. *Stroke* 1984; **15**: 566–570.

Study design

Class of evidence	II
Randomization	None (see below)
Number of patients	3521 (2922 had aneurysm surgery)
Length of follow-up	6 months
Number of centres	68 in 14 countries (24 in USA)
Stratification	Age
	Sex
	Presence of hypertension
	Site and size of aneurysm

- ◆ Aim of the study was two-fold; firstly to define the relationship between timing of aneurysm surgery and outcome, secondly to document current medical and surgical management in a number of centres around the world.
- ◆ It was a prospective, observational, epidemiological survey.
- ◆ Assessments were performed by a neurologist and blinded to the timing of surgery.

- All patients admitted to each participant centre were enrolled, with four 'logs' completed for each—'SAH log', 'registration form', 'treatment form', and 'follow-up form'.
- Inclusion criteria: Admission ≤3 days since first SAH from a saccular aneurysm (computed tomography scan/lumbar puncture (CT/LP), confirmation of bleed, angio/surgical confirmation of aneurysm).
- Exclusion criteria: Delayed admission >3 days since bleed; multiple bleeds; no confirmation of aneurysm.
- A large number of patients were excluded for other reasons such as evacuation of haematoma, non-participating surgeon, lack of patient/carer consent etc. but these are not listed as exclusion criteria *per se*.

Outcome measures

Primary endpoints

- 'Good result' or death as defined by the Glasgow Outcome Scale (GOS)
- Neurological examination

Secondary endpoints

- Pre-, intra-, and post-operative complications

Results

Many demographic results including the age, sex, site, and size of the aneurysm(s), and the presence of pre-existing hypertension are reported in the results. In 51% of patients, surgery was performed on day 0–3. About 75–80% of patients were considered in 'good condition' at the time of admission but at 6 months, only 58% had recovered to their premorbid state without neurological deficit. Nine percent were moderately disabled, 5% severely disabled, 2% vegetative, and 26% died. Leading causes of death or disability, in descending order, were vasospasm (13.5%), direct effect of the bleed on brain parenchyma (10.6%), re-bleeding (7.5%), operative complications (4%), intracerebral haemorrhage (2%), hydrocephalus (1.7%), and other less common causes.

The most important results are probably the prognostic factors, as determined by a univariate analysis. These included:

- Level of consciousness ($p < 0.001$): 75% who were alert on admission had a good recovery, compared to 11% who were comatose
- Age inversely related to outcome (26% between 70 and 87 years had a good outcome)
- No significant sex differences
- Smaller aneurysms (<12 mm) had more favourable results
- Outcome better if middle cerebral or internal carotid aneurysm (compared to vertebrobasilar or anterior circulation)

- Other good prognostic indicators included lower admission blood pressure, clot distribution on CT, absence of pre-existing medical conditions, absence of vasospasm, admission motor response, and orientation.

In addition to these results, a number of medical conditions such as pneumonia, cardiac disturbances, gastrointestinal (GI) bleeding etc. were identified to commonly occur after admission. There was considerable difference in outcome and mortality (death ranged from 0% to 66%) between centres—Chi squared test determined that this was not related to activity of the individual centres.

Surgical results

- At 6 months, 69% who had surgery had a good result, versus 14% dead. Compare this to the 58% good recovery overall. This effect was strongly related to age (90% good result in the 18–29 years age group versus 56% in the 60–69 years age group). Factors associated with good surgical outcome were similar to the overall prognostic factors.
- Patients who were alert pre-operatively had a more favourable prognosis (overall) if their operation occurred between days 0–3 or after day 10. Operatively mortality, however, only reduced after day 10.
- Patients who were drowsy pre-operatively had better outcomes when operated after day 10.

Conclusions

The main conclusions are that 75% of those admitted within 3 days were in good condition, with a 58% good recovery at 6 months, and 25% death rate. Vasospasm and re-bleeding were the major causes of death or disability, aside from the initial effects of the bleed. There were a number of prognostic factors including admission Glasgow coma scale (GCS) and age. The study concluded that there is considerable room for improvement.

Critique

This study was performed at a time when most neurosurgeons opted to wait several days after an SAH before operating. At this point, there was little doubt that operative results were better—the patient was medically stable, and the brain was less swollen and friable. The study was really a response to the question of whether the overall management results were better i.e. by delaying surgery, some patients would suffer re-bleeds and others may suffer vasospasm that cannot be adequately treated in the presence of an unsecured aneurysm. The study also sought to look at the epidemiological and prognostic factors in these patients, and was the largest study of its time. In this sense, the study was a well-designed epidemiological study and served as a preliminary to randomized controlled trials (although these came over 20 years later). Perhaps one of the criticisms of the study is the length of follow-up, which was limited to 6 months. Patients with neurological deficits can still show improvement after this time, although the differences from a longer follow-up would probably be small.

This study had a very large impact on the management of patients with suspected aneurysmal SAH. It confirmed that patients with poor grade and older age, with pre-existing medical conditions have a very poor prognosis, and that these patients should not be operated on before day 10. It also had a profound effect on the timing of surgery of good grade patients, prompting an international change in practice to early surgery by day 3. The main difference today is that we now have the option of endovascular treatment. This is often performed on poorer grade patients within the vasospastic period, largely because it is less risky to do so. However, as a large number of aneurysms are still treated surgically, this study still has great relevance.

The timing of intervention for aneurysmal subarachnoid haemorrhage remains controversial. Of particular note is a series of 391 patients from the Alfred Hospital in Melbourne who underwent surgery within 24 h following their initial bleed (Laidlaw and Siu, 2002). In this series, 83% of patients with good clinical grades had good outcomes with early surgery. In addition, in this case series, only 15% of patients with poor clinical grades had a poor outcome.

Laidlaw JD, Siu KH. Ultra-early surgery for aneurismal subarachnoid hemorrhage: outcomes for a consecutive series of 391 patients not selected by grade or age. *J Neurosurg* 2002; **97**: 250–258.

1.2 **Endovascular coiling versus aneurysm clipping in ruptured aneurysms**

Details of study

The ISAT (International Subarachnoid Aneurysm Trial) is the most comprehensive study comparing endovascular to surgical treatment in ruptured aneurysms. It has had a greater impact on treatment of ruptured aneurysms than any other study to date.

Study references

There is an initial study with 1-year follow-up looking at primary endpoints and several 'spin-offs' looking at secondary outcome measures.

Main study

Molyneux A, Kerr R, Stratton I, Sandercock P, Clarke M, Shrimpton J, Holman R; International Subarachnoid Aneurysm Trial (ISAT) Collaborative Group. International Subarachnoid Aneurysm Trial (ISAT) of neurosurgical clipping versus endovascular coiling in 2143 patients with ruptured intracranial aneurysms: a randomised trial. Lancet 2002; **360**: 1267–1274.

Related studies

Molyneux A, Kerr R; International Subarachnoid Aneurysm Trial (ISAT) Collaborative Group, Stratton I, Sandercock P, Clarke M, Shrimpton J, Holman R. International Subarachnoid Aneurysm Trial (ISAT) of neurosurgical clipping versus endovascular coiling in 2143 patients with ruptured intracranial aneurysms: a randomized trial. *J Stroke Cerebrovasc Dis* 2002; **11**: 304–314.

Molyneux AJ, Kerr RS, Yu LM, Clarke M, Sneade M, Yarnold JA, Sandercock P; International Subarachnoid Aneurysm Trial (ISAT) Collaborative Group. International subarachnoid aneurysm trial (ISAT) of neurosurgical clipping versus endovascular coiling in 2143 patients with ruptured intracranial aneurysms: a randomised comparison of effects on survival, dependency, seizures, rebleeding, subgroups, and aneurysm occlusion. *Lancet* 2005; **366**: 809–817.

National Study of Subarachnoid Haemorrhage. Royal College of Surgeons of England, 2004.

Wolstenholme J, Rivero-Arias O, Gray A, Molyneux AJ, Kerr RS, Yarnold JA, Sneade M; International Subarachnoid Aneurysm Trial (ISAT) Collaborative Group. Treatment pathways, resource use, and costs of endovascular coiling versus surgical clipping after a SAH. *Stroke* 2008; **39**: 111–119.

Study design

- ◆ Placebo-controlled randomized trial (PRCT)

Class of evidence	I
Randomization	Non-blinded coiling versus clipping
Number of patients	2143 (1073 coiled, 1070 clipped)
Length of follow-up	Primary outcomes: 1 year
	Secondary outcomes: ongoing
Number of centres	43 (centres treating 60–200 cases per year)
Stratification	Age
	Sex
	World Federation of Neurosurgeons grade (WFNS)
	Aneurysm size and location
	Extent of blood on CT scan

- Patients were randomized after admission to a neurosurgical unit and after initial angiography. Out of 9559 patients assessed for eligibility, 2143 were deemed suitable for randomization.
- Inclusion criteria: SAH within 28 days (CT or LP proven); presence of aneurysm (proven by computed tomography angiogram (CTA) or formal angiogram); good enough clinical state to justify treatment; aneurysms judged to be suitable for either technique (opinion of both surgeon and neuroradiologist) with equipoise regarding which method would be best; consent.
- Exclusion criteria: More than 28 days since SAH; clinical condition considered unsuitable for either or both treatments; lack of consent; participation in another SAH trial.

Outcome measures

Primary endpoints

- Incidence of death or dependency; modified Rankin score

Secondary endpoints

- Subgroups—WFNS grade at randomization, age, Fischer grade, lumen size of aneurysm, aneurysm site
- Incidence of re-bleeding from the treated aneurysm
- Quality of life at 1 year
- Frequency of epilepsy
- Cost-effectiveness
- Neuropsychological outcomes
- Results of follow-up angiography

Results

About 23.7% of patients who underwent endovascular coiling were dependent or dead at 1 year compared to 30.6% who had their aneurysm surgically clipped ($p < 0.002$). This led to a relative/absolute risk reduction of dependency or death at 1 year of 22.6%/6.9% respectively. Re-bleeding risk at 1 year was 2 per 1276 patient-years in the endovascular group versus 0 per 1081 patient-years in the surgical group (not significant).

Outcome		Endovascular	Surgical
Incidence of death or dependence (mRS 3–6)		23.5%	30.9%
Mortality at 1 year		85	105
Incidence of re-bleeding (fatality in brackets)	Before treatment	17(7)	28(19)
	Re-bleed <1 year	45(22)	39(24)
	Re-bleed >1 year	7(2)	2(2)
Re-treatment rate	<1 year	121	32
	>1 year	15	1
Complete occlusion at first follow-up angiography		66%	82%
Incidence of seizures		60	112

Conclusions

The outcome, in terms of survival-free disability, is significantly better with endovascular treatment than with surgical clipping of a ruptured aneurysm.

Critique

There is no doubt that the ISAT trial has generated a large amount of controversy among neurosurgeons and interventional radiologists alike. Whatever the criticism, it is one of the few multi-centre, randomized trials in neurosurgery and most would admit that it is of considerable importance. However, some have argued that the results have been over-interpreted. One of the major criticisms is that it compares good interventional neuro-radiologists to 'average' neurosurgeons rather than those who 'concentrate' on neurovascular surgery. In other words, there is an inherent bias in the recruiting centres as being those that have a strong interventional radiology interest. The ISAT group have countered this by stating that the trial is a 'pragmatic' trial. That is, it tries to determine the best outcome for a patient, in a real life situation who would be transferred to their regional unit for diagnosis and treatment. It is not a trial of 'the best possible surgery versus the best possible endovascular treatment' but a trial of what the best option is for an 'average patient'.

A second criticism of the trial is the randomization process. The trial is biased towards small anterior circulation aneurysms (97.5%). To be fair, the ISAT investigators have never claimed that the trial indicates that all ruptured aneurysms should be coiled in preference to clipping. But some people have perhaps interpreted it thus. Also concerned with the randomization process is that the average time to randomization was slightly longer in the surgical group (1.7 versus 1.1 days) and this may have led to slightly worse outcomes in this group. Since the numbers of re-bleeds takes into account those that happen after randomization but before treatment, this may have led to a worsening of results in the surgical group.

Since the analysis is based on an intention-to-treat paradigm, some patients allocated endovascular treatment received clipping (for a variety of reasons, including patient choice) and 38 allocated clipping crossed over to the endovascular group. However, the analysis is based on the original randomization choice and this has received some criticism in the literature.

Probably the most important criticism of the ISAT trial is that the primary endpoints were measured at 1 year and not subsequently. Therefore, the trial shows that in the initial phase, endovascular may be better than surgical treatment. But does this necessarily translate into the long term? There is some evidence from early analysis of the secondary data that in fact the surgical group may just be slower to recover and that there is some improvement in modified Rankin score (mRS) with time. Also, there is the issue of long-term re-bleed rates. The late re-bleed rate in the endovascular group is 0.21% per patient-year compared to 0.063% in the surgical group. This coupled with the fact that the poor outcome at 1 year is much less than in the surgical group of patients less than 40 years of age has led some ISAT investigators to suggest that surgery may be better in this age group.

Whatever the criticisms, ISAT has provided a wealth of useful data that will continue to be analysed for years to come. Many follow-up studies are expected, including cognitive and neuropsychological outcomes, long-term re-bleed rates, and long-term re-treatment rates. The trial has led to a huge shift from surgery to endovascular treatment in some centres, particularly in the UK and France. Time will tell whether this shift has been appropriate.

1.3 Long-term natural history of unruptured aneurysms

Details of study

The International Study of Unruptured Intracranial Aneurysms (ISUIA) was the first large-scale, prospective study looking at the natural history of unruptured aneurysms as well as the risks of treatment of unruptured aneurysms. Factors related to prognosis are elucidated.

Study references

Main study

International Study of Unruptured Intracranial Aneurysms Investigators. Unruptured intracranial aneurysms: natural history, clinical outcome, and risks of surgical and endovascular treatment. *Lancet* 2003; **362**: 103–110.

Related study

'ISUIA 1' (a retrospective study):

International Study of Unruptured Intracranial Aneurysms Investigators. Unruptured intracranial aneurysms – risk of rupture and risks of surgical intervention. *N Engl J Med* 1998; **339**: 1725–1733.

Study design

This is a natural history study including 4060 patients from 61 centres worldwide. Eligible patients were prospectively identified by study investigators. Patients were assigned to either an unoperated or operated cohort, depending on whether operative treatment (open or endovascular) was intended. Unoperated patients were then divided into two groups. The study looked at unruptured aneurysms that were either associated with no previous subarachnoid haemorrhage from a separate aneurysm (Group 1) or previous subarachnoid haemorrhage from a separate aneurysm (Group 2). A second objective was to look at factors that increased risk. In the operated cohort, the objective was to look at treatment morbidity and mortality. All patients underwent angiography.

- Inclusion criteria: Greater than or equal to 1 unruptured intracranial saccular aneurysm (regardless of symptoms other than rupture, e.g. cranial nerve palsy); Rankin 1 or 2 (self-caring) after previous rupture (patients may not have had previous rupture).

- Exclusion criteria: Fusiform, mycotic, or traumatic aneurysms; aneurysm <2 mm; SAH from single ruptured aneurysm or unknown source; unruptured aneurysm that was manipulated prior to study; previous intracranial haemorrhage of unknown cause or untreated structural abnormality; malignant brain tumour; bedridden or unable to communicate when aneurysm identified.

Outcome measures

- Subarachnoid haemorrhage and size of aneurysm were the most important factors in the unoperated cohort.
- Death and disability were the most important factors in the operated cohort.

Results

Five-year cumulative rupture rates (5 YRR)

- Less than 7 mm aneurysms

	Cumulative 5 YRR	
	Group 1	Group 2
Cavernous carotid artery aneurysms	0	0
A.comm or ACA aneurysms	0	1–5%
Vertebrobasilar, PCA or P.comm aneurysms	2–5%	3–4%

- 7–12 mm aneurysms

	Cumulative 5 YRR
Cavernous carotid artery aneurysms	0
A.comm or ACA aneurysms	2–6%
Vertebrobasilar, PCA or P.comm aneurysms	14.5%

- Greater than 12 mm aneurysms

	Cumulative 5 YRR	
	13–24 mm	>25 mm
Cavernous carotid artery aneurysms	3.0%	6.4%
A.comm or ACA aneurysms	15.5%	40%
Vertebrobasilar, PCA or P.comm aneurysms	18.4%	50%

Conditions that led to diagnosis did not differ significantly between cohorts. Fifty-one patients (3%) in the unoperated cohort had a rupture, of which 49 occurred within 5 years. For patients with aneurysms less than 7 mm, groups 1 and 2 were significantly different ($p < 0.0001$). In summary, Group 1 (no previous SAH from a separate aneurysm) had a lower risk of rupture than Group 2. Rupture rate was dependent on location; the greatest risk being associated with posterior circulation aneurysms. For larger aneurysms, there was no significant difference between groups, but rupture was also related to size and location and reached 50% over 5 years for vertebrobasilar, posterior cerebral artery (PCA), or posterior communicating artery (P.comm) aneurysms greater than 25 mm. Multivariate analysis showed that age was not a factor.

In the craniotomy part of the surgical cohort, risks associated with treatment included age >50 years, diameter >12 mm, location in posterior circulation, previous ischaemic cerebrovascular disease and aneurysmal symptoms other than rupture. In the endovascular group, diameter > 12 mm and posterior circulation only were associated with poor outcome. Overall mortality and morbidity was between 7.1% and 12.6% depending on group and cohort.

Conclusions

Aneurysmal rupture rate is related to size and location of aneurysm and for aneurysms <7 mm, risk is increased with previous SAH from a separate aneurysm. These factors, coupled with the morbidity/mortality data allow neurosurgeons to make an informed choice on whether to operate or not. In general, the risk of rupture for a particular aneurysm over the patient's remaining lifetime can be compared to the mortality/morbidity risk.

Critique

The ISUIA was a prospective study of over 4000 patients and as such is the best natural history study to date. The main limitations (as cited in the study) include the non-randomized nature of the surgical versus non-surgical cohorts, the variable follow-up that was less than 5 years in over 50% of the patients, and the relatively low numbers in the endovascular cohort. Furthermore, the low numbers recruited from each centre have led some critics to suggest that the total numbers represent less than 10% of patients (on average) from each centre. This implies an inherent selection bias. Another criticism is that there were substantial differences between the patients in the untreated versus the treated groups. For example, the untreated group had a higher incidence of prior SAH, cerebrovascular disease, intracranial haemorrhage, transient ischaemic attack, hypertension and its treatment, myocardial infarction, and alcohol and tobacco abuse. The same group had lower rates of cranial nerve deficit, mass effect, seizures, headaches, CT or magnetic resonance imaging (MRI) diagnosis, family history, and use of oral contraceptives or stimulants. In the 'no treatment' group, 36 cases of SAH due to another (undetermined) potential source of haemorrhage were excluded. No analysis of aneurysm shape or the presence of daughter sacs were included in the study.

Despite criticisms regarding selection bias, ISUIA has had a profound impact on the decision to treat unruptured aneurysms. Whilst some have relied on its interpretation more than others, it has provided an invaluable additional tool to neurosurgeons and interventionalists alike.

1.4 **Nimodipine for prophylaxis of cerebral vasospasm in aneurysmal subarachnoid haemorrhage**

Details of study

The 'British Aneurysm Nimodipine Trial' was one of the first properly randomized trials involving neurosurgical patients. It showed reduced cerebral infarction and better outcome in patients given nimodipine.

Study references

Main reference

Pickard JD, Murray GD, Illingworth R, Shaw MDM, Teasdale GM, Foy PM, Humphrey PRD, Lang DA, Nelson R, Richards P, Sinar J, Bailey S, Skene A. Effect of oral nimodipine on cerebral infarction and outcome after subarachnoid haemorrhage: British aneurysm nimodipine trial. *BMJ* 1989; **298**: 636–642.

Related references

Allen GS, Ahn HS, Preziosi TJ, Battye R, Boone SC, Boone SC, Chou SN, Kelly DL, Weir BK, Crabbe RA, Lavik PJ, Rosenbloom SB, Dorsey FC, Ingram CR, Mellits DE, Bertsch LA, Boisvert DP, Hundley MB, Johnson RK, Strom JA, Transou CR. Cerebral arterial spasm – a controlled trial of nimodipine in patients with subarachnoid hemorrhage. *N Engl J Med* 1983; **308**: 619–624.

Barker FG, Ogilvy CS. Efficacy of prophylactic nimodipine for delayed ischaemic deficit after subarachnoid hemorrhage: a meta-analysis. *J Neurosurg* 1996; **84**: 405–414.

Dorhout Mees SM, Rinkel GJE, Feigin VL, Algra A, van den Bergh WM, Vermeulen M, van Gijn N. Calcium antagonists for subarachnoid haemorrhage. *Cochrane database of systematic reviews* 2007, Issue 3. Art no.: CD000277. DOI: 10.1002/14651858.CD000277.pub3.

Study design

◆ Double blind, PRCT

Class of evidence	I
Randomization	Nimodipine versus placebo
Number of patients	554 total
Length of follow-up	3 months
Number of centres	4
Stratification	A subgroup stratification compared prognostic factors in the two groups, including age, sex, loss of consciousness at ictus, time from haemorrhage to entry, GCS, limb weakness, neck stiffness, hypertension, angiographic, and CT findings

◆ Aim was to determine if 60 mg oral nimodipine 4-hourly reduces the incidence of cerebral ischaemia and infarction arising *de novo* after spontaneous aneurysmal subarachnoid haemorrhage.

- The main distinction in outcome was between moderate or good outcome and poor outcome i.e. death or severe disability.
- Treatment started within 96 h of haemorrhage and continued for 21 days.
- Demographic data and clinical data including past medical history and status on admission (including WFNS grade) were also recorded.
- Inclusion Criteria: Greater than or equal to 96 h since bleed (SAH proven by CT or LP); >18 years of age.
- Exclusion criteria: Less than or equal to 96 h since bleed; major co-morbidities (renal, hepatic, pulmonary, and cardiac disease); coma due to SAH within the week prior to latest SAH; lack of consent.

Outcome measures

Primary endpoints

- Rate of cerebral infarction, re-bleed or poor outcome between the two groups

Secondary endpoints

- Glasgow Outcome Score (scale of 1 to 5) at least 3 months after haemorrhage

Other secondary outcomes were causes of disability or death, including initial bleed, ischaemia, re-bleed, intracranial haematoma, hydrocephalus, operative complications, and other/unknown causes.

Results

Follow-up at 3 months showed that 21 days of nimodipine treatment was effective in reducing the incidence of cerebral infarction by one-third (22% with nimodipine compared to 33% with placebo). This constitutes a reduction of 34% or 37% of definite infarcts ($p = 0.014$). Poor outcomes reduced significantly by 40% with nimodipine compared to placebo (20% versus 33% respectively, $p < 0.001$). Certain factors were individually, but not independently, associated with better outcome but there was no evidence that benefit from treatment was confined to any particular subgroup. There was no significant effect on mortality between the groups.

Conclusions

Oral nimodipine 60 mg 4-hourly is well tolerated and reduces cerebral infarction and improves outcome after subarachnoid haemorrhage.

Critique

The first randomized, double-blind, placebo-controlled trial of nimodipine was reported in 1983 (Allen *et al.*, 1983). The authors evaluated the prophylactic use of nimodipine for 21 days following aneurysmal SAH in 125 patients of good grade and found that nimodipine was effective in reducing neurological deficits. This study by Pickard *et al.* reported in 1989 is the largest RCT that evaluated a calcium antagonist and included 554 SAH patients. The demographic and clinical data between the treated and placebo groups are not significantly different. However, there was an increased prevalence of hypertension, neck stiffness and non-reactive pupils in the nimodipine group. These factors are generally associated with poor prognosis and therefore the fact that the nimodipine group did better would suggest that, if anything, the results are under-representative of any difference. By contrast, the placebo group had a larger number of patients with pre-existing cardiovascular disease and smokers. A second criticism relates to the age of the study. In the late 1980s, the usual treatment for aneurysm rupture was surgical clipping. In this trial, 187 and 181 patients in each group had proven aneurysms on angiography. Therefore, this trial is not confined to treated aneurysmal subarachnoid haemorrhage nor does it include endovascular treatment. It does however suggest that nimodipine is important in the early stages after subarachnoid haemorrhage though the 21-day limit is somewhat arbitrary. This landmark trial has led to virtually every subarachnoid haemorrhage patient being given nimodipine, worldwide. At least five other RCTs of prophylactic nimodipine have been carried out and a meta-analysis concluded that the effectiveness of nimodipine had been well demonstrated and supported routine prophylactic nimodipine administration (Barker *et al.*, 1996). Although other calcium antagonists, such as nicardipine, have been investigated, a systematic review of 27 RCTs concluded that there was only evidence to support the prophylactic use of nimodipine (Dorhout Mees *et al.*, 2007).

Barker FG, Ogilvy CS. Efficacy of prophylactic nimodipine for delayed ischaemic deficit after subarachnoid hemorrhage: a meta-analysis. *J Neurosurg* 1996; **84**: 405–414.

Dorhout Mees SM, Rinkel GJE, Feigin VL, Algra A, van den Bergh WM, Vermeulen M, van Gijn N. Calcium antagonists for subarachnoid haemorrhage. *Cochrane database of systematic reviews* 2007, Issue 3. Art no.: CD000277. DOI: 10.1002/14651858.CD000277.pub3.

1.5 'HHH' therapy for vasospasm

Details of study

Kassell and co. carried out a large study in 1982 to evaluate the effects of hypertensive therapy and intravascular volume expansion in a series of 58 patients with delayed ischaemic neurological deficits (DINDs) following aneurysmal subarachnoid haemorrhage. This was the first large series to examine the role of hypertension and hypervolaemia to treat neurological deficits due to vasospasm following subarachnoid haemorrhage.

Study references

Main study

Kassell NF, Peerless SJ, Durwood QJ, Beck DW, Drake CG, Adams HP. Treatment of ischaemic deficits from vasospasm with intravascular volume expansion and induced arterial hypertension. *Neurosurgery* 1982; **11**: 337–343.

Related reference

Kosnik EJ, Hunt WE. Postoperative hypertension in the management of patients with intracranial arterial aneurysms. *J Neurosurg* 1976; **45**: 148–154.

Study design

This study was a retrospective series analysis of 58 patients with neurological deficits and proven angiographic vasospasm in whom arterial hypertension was induced in an attempt to reverse the neurological deficits.

Treatment protocol

The protocol for inducing hypertension and volume expansion evolved throughout the series but included the use of transfusion of blood and blood products, the use of colloids, and administration of vasopressors if necessary. Fludrocortisone was also administered to help maintain hypervolaemia. Target parameters included a central venous pressure (CVP) of 10 mmHg and pulmonary artery wedge pressure (PAWP) of 18–20 mmHg. Estimates were made on an individual patient basis as to the systolic pressure that would likely be required to reverse the neurological deficits. Once deficit reversal was achieved the systolic pressure was kept at the minimum level required to sustain deficit reversal. Maximal systolic parameters were set at 240 mmHg systolic in patients with secured aneurysms and at 160 mmHg in unsecured aneurysms.

Results

◆ Mean age of patients was 51 years.

◆ Twenty-two patients had unsecured aneurysms at the time of induced hypertension.

Clinical outcomes

Permanent improvement in neurological deficit	74%
No change in deficits	16%
Deterioration	10%
Most common complications	Aneurysmal re-bleed (19%) Pulmonary oedema (17%)
Most common cause of treatment failure	Established infarction (17%)

- Kassell *et al.* reported that reversal of deficits was seen within 1 h in 81% and that the period of induced-hypertension varied between 12 h and 8 days.
- Other complications included dilutional hypernatraemia, coagulopathy, haemothorax, and myocardial infarction.

Conclusions

- Hypertension and hypervolaemia are relatively safe and effective in reversing neurological deficits due to vasospasm in patients with subarachnoid haemorrhage.
- Hypertension/hypervolaemia is most effective for patients with mild deficits.

Critique

DIND is a major cause of morbidity and mortality following aneurysmal SAH. Kosnik and Hunt were the first to report the effects of raising arterial pressure in cerebral vasospasm (Kosnik and Hunt, 1974). They reported a series of seven patients in whom the neurological deficit was reversed promptly by the elevation of systemic blood pressure and found that infarction was prevented in some of these patients. Kassell and co. carried out the larger study considered here that showed that hypertensive therapy and intravascular volume expansion resulted in sustained neurological benefits in the majority of patients. One of the most significant observations of Kassell and co.'s study was that hypertension and hypervolaemia were most effective in patients with mild deficits and that these could be anticipated in patients between days 5 and 12 post-bleed who had large blood loads on their CT scans. Although they recommended angiography to confirm the presence of spasm they also maintained that if angiography was not accessible then a diagnosis of vasospasm could be made presumptively by excluding other causes of neurological deterioration such as re-bleed or hydrocephalus.

Since these early studies, HHH therapy has evolved to include haemodilution to augment rheological properties of blood flow. Although HHH therapy has not been examined with a randomized controlled trial, it has become the mainstay of medical therapy for the treatment of vasospasm. Recent investigations using cerebral monitoring support its continued use on the basis of improved physiological parameters at least (Raabe *et al.*, 2005). There is no consensus as to how HHH therapy should be achieved although high-dependency care with invasive cardiovascular monitoring is commonly employed.

HHH therapy is not without risks and is associated with significant complications including pulmonary oedema, myocardial ischaemia, and electrolyte abnormalities including dilutional hyponatraemia. The prophylactic use of HHH therapy has not been widely supported and preliminary trials have not shown any benefits (Solenksi *et al.*, 1995; Solomen *et al.*, 1998). It is to be expected that in the coming years functional imaging modalities and invasive cerebral tissue monitoring may lead to refinements in the optimization of cerebral perfusion augmentation therapy.

Raabe A, Beck J, Keller M, Vatter H, Zimmermann M, Seifert V. Relative importance of hypertension compared with hypervolemia for increasing cerebral oxygenation in patients with cerebral vasospasm after subarachnoid hemorrhage. *J Neurosurg* 2005; **103**: 974–981.

Solenski NJ, Haley EC Jr, Kassell NF, Kongable G, Germanson T, Truslowski L and Torner JC. Medical complications of subarachnoid haemorrhage: a report of the multicentre, cooperative aneurysm study. Participants of the Multicentre Cooperative Aneurysm Study. *Crit Care Med* 1995; **23**: 1007–1017.

Solomon RA, Fink ME, Lennihan L. Prophylactic volume expansion therapy for the prevention of delayed cerebral ischaemia after early aneurysm surgery. Results of a preliminary trial. *Arch Neurol* 1988; **45**: 325–332.

1.6 **Statins in the prevention of vasospasm in aneurysmal subarachnoid haemorrhage**

Details of study

While there has been evidence of the beneficial effects of statins in subarachnoid haemorrhage prior to 2005, this study is the first randomized, phase II trial and looks specifically at the effect of pravastatin on patient outcome in subarachnoid haemorrhage.

Study references

There is an initial study with immediate follow-up looking at primary endpoints, followed by a number of other papers looking at extended (6-month) follow-up and other effects of pravastatin. The outcome of this trial has led to a much larger phase III trial of simvastatin that is underway at the time of writing (the 'STASH' trial).

Main study

Tseng MY, Czosnyka M, Richards H, Pickard JD, Kirkpatrick PJ. Effects of acute treatment with pravastatin on cerebral vasospasm, autoregulation, and delayed ischemic deficits after aneurysmal subarachnoid hemorrhage: a phase II randomized placebo-controlled trial. *Stroke* 2005; **36**: 1627–1632.

Related references

Lynch JR, Wang H, McGirt MJ, Floyd J, Friedman AH, Coon AL, Blessing R, Alexanderander MJ, Graffagnino C, Warner DS, Laskowitz DT. Simvastatin reduces vasospasm after aneurysmal subarachnoid hemorrhage: results of a pilot randomized clinical trial. *Stroke* 2005; **36**: 2024–2026.

Tseng MY, Hutchinson PJ, Czosnyka M, Richards H, Pickard JD, Kirkpatrick PJ. Effects of acute pravastatin treatment on intensity of rescue therapy, length of inpatient stay, and 6-month outcome in patients after aneurysmal subarachnoid hemorrhage. *Stroke* 2007; **38**: 1545–1550.

Tseng MY, Hutchinson PJ, Turner CL, Czosnyka M, Richards H, Pickard JD, Kirkpatrick PJ. Biological effects of acute pravastatin treatment in patients after aneurysmal subarachnoid hemorrhage: a double-blind, placebo-controlled trial. *J Neurosurg* 2007; **107**: 1092–1100.

Study design

- Double-blind PRCT
- This is a phase II trial looking at safety and therefore only has small numbers of patients from a single centre. Its main purpose is as a pilot study to assess whether a larger

Class of evidence	I
Randomization	Pravastatin versus placebo
Number of patients	80 (equally distributed)
Length of follow-up	Not relevant as this is a phase II trial looking at safety and immediate clinical and physiological effects (however, 6-month data are the subject of a related publication)
Number of centres	1
Stratification	None, but baseline characteristics similar in the two groups

phase III trial is needed to evaluate whether pravastatin reduces vasospasm or its consequences including delayed ischaemic deficit (DID).

- As well as primary and secondary endpoints, baseline clinical data were measured. These included age, gender, medical history, WFNS grade, and also, radiological characteristics including Fisher grade on CT, presence of hydrocephalus or intraventricular blood, location of aneurysm on angiography.
- Trial medication (pravastatin sodium 40 mg daily) was started within 72 h of ictus and continued up to 14 days or until discharge.
- The main aim was to see if pravastatin reduces vasospasm or its consequences including DID.
- Inclusion criteria: Aneurysmal SAH; age 18–84 years.
- Exclusion criteria: Non-aneurysmal SAH; pregnancy; pre-ictal statin therapy; contraindication to statins (liver or renal dysfunction, or ALT >50 U/L).

Outcome measures

Primary endpoints

- Incidence, severity, and duration of vasospasm on transcranial Doppler (TCD) indices
- Duration of impaired cerebral autoregulation

Secondary endpoints

- Evidence of vasospasm-related DIDs
- Disability at discharge

Results

Baseline characteristics of age, sex, WFNS grade, Fisher grade, hydrocephalus, intraventricular haemorrhage (IVH), or aneurysm location did not differ significantly between the two groups. Similarly, post-operative characteristics including need for extraventricular drain (EVD), ventriculitis, numbers clipped versus coiled, sepsis, or reason for end of trial (e.g. discharge or death, etc.) did not differ between the groups. There was a trend for more post-operative deficits in the pravastatin group ($p = 0.115$) but a trend for more deaths in the placebo group (again, not significant).

	Placebo	Pravastatin group	Degree of change	Statistical significance
Vasospasm on TCD	25%	17%	−32%	$p = 0.006$
Severe vasospasm	12%	7%	−42%	$p = 0.044$
Duration of severe vasospasm	1.2 days	0.5 days	−0.8 days	$p = 0.068$
Period of impaired ipsilateral cerebral autoregulation	5.3 days	3 days	−2.4 days	$p = 0.011$

In the placebo group, there was a reduction in both primary endpoints with a 32% reduction in vasospasm on TCD in the pravastatin group ($p = 0.006$) and a 42% reduction in severe vasospasm ($p = 0.044$). The duration of vasospasm was shortened by 0.8 days in the pravastatin group ($p = 0.068$). The period of impaired cerebral autoregulation was shorter with pravastatin (ipsilateral side by 2.4 days, $p = 0.011$). With regard to the secondary endpoints, the incidence of vasospasm-related DIDs was 83% reduced in the pravastatin group ($p < 0.001$). Pravastatin was associated with a reduction in disability at discharge and a reduction in mortality of 75% ($p = 0.037$). Subsequent follow-up shows that these beneficial effects were still present at 6 months (Tseng et al., 2007).

Conclusions

Immediate statin therapy reduces potentially adverse physiological and clinical events after an acute cerebrovascular illness.

Critique

Previous studies evaluating the role of statins in the prevention of cerebral vasospasm were retrospective, observational studies. Earlier studies had reported differences in outcome between patients already taking statins and those not on anticholesterol medications. This small randomized study by Tseng et al. with pravastatin reported in 2005 demonstrated a reduced incidence of vasospasm in patients treated with pravastatin. The pravastatin incidence of TCD-detected vasospasm was reduced by 32% with a reduced incidence of DIND and mortality. At 6 months, beneficial effects on physical and psychological aspects of functioning have subsequently been reported. Lynch et al. also reported the results of a smaller randomized clinical trial of simvastatin (Lynch et al., 2005). Their study included simvastatin versus placebo randomly allocated to 39 patients within 48 h of the SAH ictus and they reported a reduction in vasospasm in those receiving simvastatin ($p < 0.05$). Vasospasm was defined by clinical impression in the presence of at least one confirmatory radiological test (TCD or angiography). The study was not powered to answer the definitive question as to whether simvastatin was effective in reducing vasospasm, but the authors were able to conclude that simvastatin was safe and well tolerated in subarachnoid patients. Both the simvastatin study by Lynch et al. and the pravastatin study by Tseng et al. were randomized, placebo-controlled trials, making them valuable contributors to the question of whether statins are beneficial in aneurysmal subarachnoid haemorrhage. They are examples of how even small, simple studies can provide essential evidence that can lead to larger, multi-centre trials to answer a simple clinical question. The authors do not purport to show improved clinical outcome but rather look at short-term DIDs and, by measuring transcranial Doppler blood flows between the two groups, attempt to provide a pathophysiological reason for the improvement. In this sense, both studies make the assumption that TCDs are a good indicator of cerebral blood flow and that improvements in TCDs are the reasons for the improved outcome. Like any good 'pilot' studies, certain questions are left unanswered.

Another restriction of the pravastatin trial is the relatively small number of aneurysms treated with coil embolization, as compared to clipping. Although pravastatin had the same effect on both groups, the coil embolization group was small and this is essentially a trial of pravastatin in aneurysms that were surgically clipped. This will be resolved by the larger multi-centre study. Another question raised in the literature is the increased rate of sepsis, including ventriculitis, in the pravastatin group. Although this did not reach significance, and did not appear to contribute to a worse mortality, it will need to be addressed in a larger trial. The pravastatin trial has led to a multi-centre randomized controlled trial looking at the potential benefit of simvastatin (40 mg for 21 days) in aneurysmal SAH (STASH) that is underway. Some centres have already routinely started using statins in SAH.

Lynch JR, Wang H, McGirt MJ, Floyd J, Friedman AH, Coon AL, Blessing R, Alexanderander MJ, Graffagnino C, Warner DS, Laskowitz DT. Simvastatin reduces vasospasm after aneurysmal subarachnoid hemorrhage: results of a pilot randomized clinical trial. *Stroke* 2005; **36**: 2024–2026.

1.7 **Treatment of cerebral arteriovenous malformations**
Details of studies

Predicting the risks of treatment is difficult due to the heterogeneity of AVMs, which vary from 'simple' to 'complex'. Spetzler and Martin reported a six-tier grading system that they retrospectively applied to a series of 100 AVMs (Spetzler and Martin, 1986). Hamilton and Spetzler subsequently validated this grading system prospectively in a series of 120 consecutive patients (Hamilton and Spetzler, 1994). The main findings of these landmarks studies have been summarized and considered here.

Study reference

Main studies

Spetzler RF, Martin NA. A proposed grading system for arteriovenous malformations. *J Neurosurgery* 1986; **65**: 476–483.

Hamilton MG, Spetzler RF. The prospective application of a grading system for arteriovenous malformations. *Neurosurgery* 1994; **34**: 2–6.

Related reference

Luessenhop AJ, Gennarelli TA. Anatomical grading of supratentorial arteriovenous malformations for determining operability. *Neurosurgery* 1977; **1**: 30–35.

Study design

* Spetzler and Martin, 1986: retrospective analysis of 100 patients with AVMs
* Hamilton and Spetzler, 1994: prospective analysis of 120 patients with AVMs

The grading system proposed by Spetzler and Martin is a six-tier system awarding points as follows:

Feature of AVM		Points
Size of AVM	>6 cm (large)	3
	3–6 cm (medium)	2
	<3 cm (small)	1
Eloquence of adjacent brain	Eloquent	1
	Non-eloquent	0
Pattern of venous drainage	Deep	1
	Superficial only	0

* Grade I lesions: small, superficial, and located in non-eloquent cortex
* Grade V lesions: large, deep, and located in critical neurological areas
* Grade VI lesions are considered inoperable lesions.

Results

Retrospective series (Spetzler and Martin, 1986)

- Grading of AVM correlated with results of surgery (Fig. 1.1).

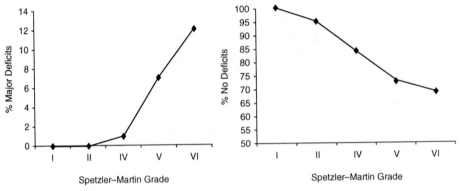

Fig. 1.1 Correlation of surgical results with Spetzler–Martin AVM grading.

Prospective series (Hamilton and Spetzler, 1994)

- Outcomes were assessed using the Glasgow Outcome Score.
- Follow-up was 77.4% at 1 year.
- Grading of AVMs was correlated with the development of both temporary ($p < 0.0001$) and permanent ($p = 0.008$) neurological deficits.
- Correlation was greatest when all three components of the grading system were applied.
- Grading of AVMs was correlated with outcome (Fig. 1.2).

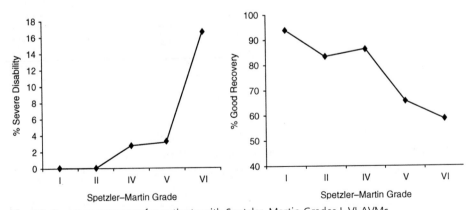

Fig. 1.2 One-year outcomes for patients with Spetzler–Martin Grades I–VI AVMs.

Conclusions

The Spetzler, Martin, and Hamilton grading system is a robust and accurate method of predicting risk of intervention in patients with AVMs.

Critique

Determination of the natural history of AVM is essential in order to assess whether the risks of surgical intervention are less than the long-term risks of conservative management. Epidemiological studies have been difficult due to heterogeneous patient populations and variation in treatment practices. Numerous studies have been carried out to address this question. Perhaps the longest prospective study to date was begun in Finland in 1965 with a 24-year follow-up of 160 patients being reported in 1990 (Troupp *et al.*, 1970; Ondra *et al.*, 1990). Two large prospective population-based studies are currently ongoing. One is the New York Islands AVM Study (NYIAVMS) (Stapf *et al.*, 2003). The other is the Scottish Intracranial Vascular Malformation Study (SIVMS) (Al-Shahi *et al.*, 2003). However, from the literature to date it appears that the risk of intracranial haemorrhage from AVMs is 1–4% per year with an annual mortality of 1–1.5%, and that the risk of bleeding of unruptured AVMs appears to be approximately 2% per year with re-bleed risk of 18% within the first year (Al-Shahi and Warlow, 2001). Surgery for AVMs is indicated only when the risk of operation is less than the risk of a conservative course of management as determined by the natural history of the AVM. The results of the NYIAVMS and SIVMS studies will be invaluable in helping determine the natural history of AVMs.

The grading system of Spetzler and Martin aimed to provide a simplified objective method of predicting the risks of surgical intervention in individual cases of AVM. Although previous grading systems had been reported they were primarily based on the AVM anatomy (Luessenhop and Gennarelli, 1977). The grading system of Spetzler and Martin takes into account the variables of vascular steal, eloquence of adjacent brain and venous drainage patterns. Their retrospective and prospective data strongly support the predictive validity of their grading scale as a robust mechanism to objectively predict outcome in individual AVMs. The greatest weakness of the study is that it was a single-centre study. However, the authors cited two other published series that had used their grading system as independent validation (Steinmeier *et al.*, 1989; Heros *et al.*, 1990). In addition, this grading system has been criticized for being over simplified. Samson and Batjer proposed that Grade IV and V AVMs might be considered as a separate entity as it is these grades that are associated with a post-operative morbidity and that a narrative description of the complexities of these AVMs might be more useful to those considering surgical intervention (Samson and Batjer, 1994). Nonetheless, the grading system developed by Spetzler, Martin, and Hamilton remains a landmark in neurovascular neurosurgery and is a useful tool for the comparison of different treatment modalities and regimes. Spetzler's group has continued to use this classification system to establish the risks and benefits of treatment of AVMs (Han *et al.*, 2003).

In addition to surgical resection, several other modalities are now available for the treatment of AVMs including endovascular techniques (Martin *et al.*, 2000) and stereotactic radiosurgery (Friedman *et al.*, 1995). However, a Cochrane Review by Al-Shahi and Warlow revealed that there are no randomized trials with clear outcomes comparing modalities (Al-Shahi and Warlow, 2006).

Al-Shahi R, Warlow C. A systematic review of the frequency and prognosis of arteriovenous malformations of the brain in adults. *Brain* 2001; **124**: 1900–1926.

Al-Shahi R, Warlow CP. Interventions for treating brain arteriovenous malformations in adults *Cochrane Database Syst Rev* 2006; **1**: CD003436.

Al-Shahi R, Bhattacharya JJ, Currie DG, Papanastassiou V, Ritchie V, Roberts RC, Sellar RJ, Warlow CP; Scottish Intracranial Vascular Malformation Study Collaborators. Prospective, population-based detection of intracranial vascular malformations in adults: the Scottish Intracranial Vascular Malformation Study (SIVMS). *Stroke* 2003; **34**: 1163–1169.

Friedman WA, Bova FJ, Mendenhall WM. Linear accelerator radiosurgery for arteriovenous malformations: the relationship of size to outcome. *J Neurosurg* 1995; **82**: 180–189.

Han PP, Ponce FA, Spetzler RF. Intention-to-treat analysis of Spetzler-Martin grades IV and V arteriovenous malformations: natural history and treatment paradigm. *J Neurosurg* 2003; **98**: 3–7.

Heros RC, Korosue K, Diebold PM. Surgical excision of cerebral arteriovenous malformations: late results. *Neurosurgery* 1990; **26**: 570–577.

Luessenhop AJ. Gennarelli TA. Anatomical grading of supratentorial arteriovenous malformations for determining operability. *Neurosurgery* 1977; **1**: 30–35.

Martin NA, Khanna R, Doberstein C, Bentson J. Therapeutic embolisation of arteriovenous malformations: the case for and against. *Clin Neurosurg* 2000; **46**: 295–318.

Ondra S, Troupp H, George ED, Schwab K. The natural history of symptomatic arteriovenous malformations if the brain: a 24-year follow-up assessment. *J Neurosurg* 1990; **73**: 387–391.

Samson DS, Batjer HH. Grading systems for AVMs: comments. *Neurosurgery* 1994; **34**: 6–7.

Stapf C, Mast H, Sciacca RR, Berenstein A, Nelson PK, Gobin YP, Pile-Spellman J, Mohr JP; New York Islands AVM Study Collaborators. The New York Islands AVM Study: design, study progress, and initial results. *Stroke* 2003; **34**: 29–33.

Steinmeier R, Schramm J, Müller HG, Fahlbusch R. Evaluation of prognostic factors in cerebral arteriovenous malformations. *Neurosurgery* 1989; **24**: 193–200.

Troupp J, Martilla I, Halonen V. Arteriovenous malformations of the brain. Prognosis without operation. *Acta Neurochir* 1970; **22**: 125–128.

1.8 Surgery for spontaneous intracerebral haematomas

Details of study

The International Surgical Trial in Intracerebral Haemorrhage (STICH) is the largest RCT to date looking at the role of early surgery in the management of intracerebral haematomas. The study was headed by Professor Mendelow from Newcastle General Hospital and was funded by the Medical Research Council (UK). A further trial, STICH II, is now underway.

Study reference

Main study

Mendelow AD, Gregson BA, Fernandes HN, Murray GD, Teasdale GM, Hope DH, Karimi A, Shaw M, Barer DH, for the STICH investigators. Early surgery versus initial conservative treatment in patients with spontaneous supratentorial intracerebral haematomas in the International Surgical Trial in Intracerebral Haemorrhage (STICH): a randomised trial. *Lancet* 2005; **365**: 387–397.

Related references

Broderick JP. The STICH trial: what does it tell us and where do we go from here? *Stroke* 2005; **36**: 1619–1620.

Mendelow AD, Unterberg A. Surgical treatment of intracerebral haemorrhage. *Curr Opin Crit Care* 2007; **13**: 169–174.

Study design

- International multi-centre PRCT

Class of evidence	I
Randomization	Early surgery versus best medical management
Number of patients	1033 patients
Follow-up	Primary outcome: GOS at 6 months
	Secondary outcomes: Mortality at 6 months Prognosis at 6 months
	93% completed follow-up
Number of centres	83 centres in 27 countries
Stratification	According to predicted 'good' or 'poor' prognosis using a prognostic score at randomization

- Patients randomized and analysed on an intention-to-treat basis.
- Surgery was carried out within 24 h of randomization.
- Surgery included craniotomy and CT-guided aspiration of the clot and the method chosen was left to the discretion of the operating surgeon.

- The option of delayed surgery remained open to those who were randomized to the medical arm.
- 503 patients underwent early surgery and 530 patients received best medical therapy.
- Primary outcome was assessed using the 8-point GOS at 6 months.
- Inclusion criteria: CT evidence of intracerebral haematoma within 72 h; clinical uncertainty regarding the benefits of either treatment arm of the trial; haematoma diameter >2 cm; GCS ≥ 5.
- Exclusion criteria: Aneurysmal bleed; infratentorial bleed; extension of bleed into brainstem; any co-morbid factor that might interfere with outcome assessment.

Outcome measures

Primary endpoints

- GOS, Barthel index, and Rankin Scale assessed by postal questionnaire at 6 months.
- Patients with a poor prognosis at randomization were deemed to have a favourable outcome if there was a severe disability or better on the GOS.
- Patients with a good prognosis were deemed to have a favourable outcome if they had a moderate disability or better on the GOS.

Secondary endpoint

- Mortality at 6 months.

Results

Outcome	Early surgery group	Best medical management group	Statistical significance
Favourable outcome	26%	24%	None
Unfavourable outcome	74%	76%	None
Mortality	36%	37%	None

- Prognosis-based analyses did not reveal any statistically significant differences between the two arms of the trial.
- Subgroup analysis showed that a favourable outcome was more likely with early surgery for superficially based lesions (≤1 cm from cortical surface) with a 29% relative benefit but this difference was not statistically significant.

Conclusions

There is no overall benefit from early surgery versus initial conservative treatment for spontaneous supratentorial haematomas.

Critique

Patients suffering from spontaneous intracerebral haematomas represent a significant proportion of neurosurgical emergencies. Nine previous clinical trials looking at the role of surgery produced conflicting results regarding the role of surgery in the management of patients with non-aneurysmal spontaneous supratentorial haematomas. The STICH trial is the largest trial to date addressing this question. Unfortunately, STICH has been over interpreted by some to mean that there is no benefit from surgery for all supratentorial haematomas. However, STICH only looked at haematomas for which the responsible surgeon was uncertain regarding the benefits of surgery versus conservative management. The results of STICH confirm that surgeons are correct to be uncertain for these patients but the results cannot be extrapolated to all intracerebral haematomas. In STICH, the timing of surgery was relatively long after presentation (median time to surgery 30 h). There may, therefore, be a role for much earlier surgery, e.g. within 12 h of the initial bleed. In addition, most patients underwent craniotomy (77%) and so the question remains as to whether there is a role for more minimally invasive methods for evacuating haematomas.

There is a view held by some that there is a fundamental problem that needs to be addressed regarding the role of surgery in the evacuation of intracerebral haematomas—the concept of a penumbra around the clot. The rationale of clot evacuation is to control intracranial pressure (ICP) and to prevent further damage to surrounding brain. However, there is no firm evidence that there is a surrounding penumbra of brain that is at risk from the clot and more basic science needs to be done to elucidate this problem further. Certainly, the toxic effects of the clot to the surrounding brain remain to be ascertained. An alternative view to this is that preclinical animal studies may support clot evacuation and so it is reasonable to hypothesize that similar evacuation in people may have benefit. It would appear that further studies, perhaps with imaging modalities, such as fMRI or SPECT in patients with intracerebral haemorrhage (ICH) may shed more light on the natural history of intracerebral haematomas.

Although STICH has not provided a definitive answer regarding the benefit of surgery in patients with spontaneous intracerebral haematomas it has allowed the identification of possible subgroups of patients who may benefit. Three trials are currently ongoing to further evaluate this issue. STICH II is looking at surgery for lobar haemorrhage where the clot is within 1 cm of the cortical surface. CLEAR IVH is looking at whether there is a benefit for surgery to remove intraventricular clot less than 30 mL. MISTIE is looking at minimal invasive surgery to remove deep intracerebral haemorrhage.

Mendelow AD, Unterberg A. Surgical treatment of intracerebral haemorrhage. *Curr Opin Crit Care* 2007; **13**: 169–174.

1.9 **Decompressive surgery for malignant cerebral artery infarction**

Details of studies

Malignant MCA infarction (MMI) is associated with a mortality rate of 80%. Since 2000, three European trials have addressed the role of decompressive surgery in these patients: the DECIMAL trial (decompressive craniectomy in malignant MCA infarction) performed in France; the DESTINY trial (decompressive surgery for the treatment of malignant infarction of the MCA) performed in Germany; and the HAMLET trial (hemicraniectomy after MCA infarction with life-threatening oedema trial) performed in the Netherlands. Although HAMLET was still ongoing, a pooled analysis of these three trials was published in 2007. The final results of HAMLET have recently been published in 2009. In addition, a North American trial, the HeaDDFIRST trial (hemicraniectomy and durotomy on deterioration from infarction-related swelling trial), was carried out between 2000 and 2003, although this was only ever published in abstract form.

Study references

Main studies

DECIMAL trial

Vahedi K, Vicaut E, Mateo J, Kurtz A, Orabi M, Guichard JP, Boutron C, Couvreur G, Rouanet F, Touzé E, Guillon B, Carpentier A, Yelnik A, George B, Payen D, Bousser MG; DECIMAL Investigators. Sequential-design, multicenter, randomised, controlled trial of early decompressive craniectomy in malignant middle cerebral artery infarction (DECIMAL trial). *Stroke* 2007; **38**: 2506–2517.

DESTINY trial

Decompressive surgery for the treatment of malignant infarction of the middle cerebral artery (DESTINY): a randomised controlled trial. *Stroke* 2007; **38**: 2518–2525.

HAMLET trial

Hofmeijer J, Amelink GJ, Algra A, van Gijn J, Macleod MR, Kappelle LJ, van der Worp HB; HAMLET investigators. Hemicraniectomy after middle cerebral artery infarction with life-threatening edema trial (HAMLET). Protocol for a randomised controlled trial of decompressive surgery in space-occupying hemispheric infarction. *Trials* 2006; **7**: 29.

Pooled analysis of DECIMAL, DESTINY, and HAMLET trials

Vahedi, K, Hofmeijer J, Juettler E, Vicaut E, George B, Algra A, Amelink GJ, Schmiedeck P, Schwab S, Rothwell PM, Bousser MG, van der Worp HB, Hacke W, for the DECIMAL, DESTINY and HAMLET investigators. Early decompressive surgery in malignant infarction of the middle cerebral artery: a pooled analysis of three randomised trials. *Lancet Neurol* 2007; **6**: 215–222.

HeaDDFIRST trial

Frank JI. Hemicraniectomy and durotomy upon deterioration from infarction related swelling trial (HeADDFIRST): first public presentation of the primary study findings. *Neurology* 2003; **60** (Suppl 1): A426.

Related references

Carandang RA, Krieger DW. Decompressive hemicraniectomy and durotomy for malignant middle cerebral artery infarction. *Neurocrit Care* 2008; **8**: 286–289.

Gupta R, Conolly ES, Mayer S, Elkind MS. Hemicraniectomy for massive middle cerebral artery territory infarction: a systematic review. *Stroke* 2004; **35**: 539–543.

Hacke W, Schwab S, Horn M, Spranger M, DeGeorgia M, von Kummer R. 'Malignant' middle cerebral artery infarction: clinical course and prognostic signs. *Arch Neurol* 1996; **53**: 309–315.

Study design

European trials

- PRCTs

	DECIMAL	DESTINY	HAMLET
Class of evidence	I	I	I
Randomization	Surgery versus medical care	Surgery versus medical care	Surgery versus medical care
Number of patients	38	32	64
Follow-up	1 year	1 year	1 year
	Primary endpoint: Functional outcome at 6 months in survivors	Primary endpoint: Mortality at 1 month	Primary endpoint: Functional outcome (mRS score)
	Secondary endpoints: Survival at 6 and 12 months Functional outcome at 12 months	Secondary endpoints: Functional outcome at 6 and 12 months	Secondary endpoints: Case fatality Quality of life Symptoms of depression
Number of centres	13	6	6

- Inclusion criteria very similar in all trials apart from age and time allowed from onset of symptoms.

  Age: DECIMAL 18–55 years; DESTINY 18–60 years; pooled analysis of DESTINY/ DECIMAL/HAMLET 18–60 years.

  Time from onset of symptoms: DECIMAL <24 h; DESTINY <36 h; HAMLET <45 h.

- Exclusion criteria also similar: significant pre-stroke disability; significant haemorrhagic infarction; coagulopathy; poor neurological state (e.g. fixed pupils).

- MMI criteria varied slightly between trials but were defined on the basis the following criteria: clinical signs of infarction on National Institutes of Health Stroke Score (NIHSS) including a score of ≥1 for the level of consciousness; radiological (CT or MRI) documentation of unilateral MCA infarction of a predetermined percentage.
- Functional outcome defined using the modified Rankin scores and dichotomized into 'favourable' or 'good' (mRS ≤3) or 'unfavourable' or 'poor' (mRS ≥4).
- Analyses on an intention-to-treat basis in DESTINY and HAMLET.
- A sequential method of analysis applied in DECIMAL.

North American trial (HeaDDFIRST)

Class of evidence	I
Randomization	Surgery versus medical care
Number of patients	25
Follow-up	180 days
	Primary endpoint: Mortality
	Secondary endpoint: Functional outcome
Number of centres	1
Stratification	None

- Inclusion criteria: Ages 18–75; NIHSS >18; premorbid mRS <2 with complete MCA +/– ACA or PCA infarction; infarct volume >50% MCA territory or >90 cm^3 on early CT, or > 180 cm^3 on late CT.
- Randomization to surgery or medical care was triggered by development of midline shift (≥7 mm septal or >4 mm pineal gland displacement).

Pooled analysis of DECIMAL, DESTINY, and HAMLET

- Primary endpoint: mRS ≤4

Results

DECIMAL and DESTINY

- DECIMAL was discontinued early because of recruitment problems and an interim analysis indicating a significant benefit of surgery on mortality.
- Recruitment to DESTINY was discontinued early because a predetermined analysis at 6 months showed a significant benefit of surgery on mortality.

Outcomes	DECIMAL			DESTINY		
	Surgery	Medical care	Statistical significance	Surgery	Medical care	Statistical significance
'Favourable' functional outcome (mRS ≤3, 6 months)	25%	6%	None	47%	27%	None
mRS ≤4 (6 months)	65%	23%	$p = 0.01$	78%	34%	$p = 0.01$
mRS 4 (6 months)	40%	17%	$p < 0.05$	29%	7%	$p = 0.01$
Survival at 30 days	N/A	N/A	N/A	88%	47%	$p = 0.02$
Survival at 6 months	75%	22%	$p < 0.0001$	82%	47%	$p = 0.03$

- Absolute reduction in death of 52.8% with surgery in DECIMAL trial.
- There were no bedridden patients in the DECIMAL trial at the end of 12 months (mRS 5) who had undergone surgery.

Pooled analysis of DECIMAL, DESTINY, and HAMLET

Outcomes at 12 months	Surgery	Medical care	Statistical significance
Mortality	22%	71%	$p < 0.0001$
mRS 4	31%	2%	$p < 0.0001$
mRS <4	74%	23%	$p < 0.0001$

- There were no significant differences in the outcome measures between the three trials at the time of the pooled analysis.
- The absolute risk reduction (ARR) for mortality at 12 months was 51.2%.
- Seventy-five percent of survivors receiving medical care had a 'favourable' outcome (mRS <4) versus 55% of survivors who received surgery.
- Forty percent of survivors who had surgery had a moderately severe disability and were unable to walk without assistance or attend to their own bodily needs without assistance (mRS of 4) versus 8% of those who received medical care.

HAMLET

Outcomes at 1 year	Surgery	Medical care	Statistical significance
Good functional outcome (mRS ≤3)	25%	25%	None
Poor functional outcome (mRS ≥4)	75%	75%	None
Mortality	22%	59%	0.002

- Absolute risk reduction in case fatality was 38%.

HeaDDFIRST trial

Outcomes	Surgery	Medical Care	Statistical significance
Mortality at 21 days	23%	40%	$p < 0.05$
Mortality at 180 days	37.5%	40%	None

- A non-significant reduction in mortality was reported.
- Functional outcomes not reported.

Conclusions

- DECIMAL: Decompressive surgery improves survival in young patients with MMI but with an increased number of patients with moderately severe disability.
- DESTINY: Pooled analysis: Early decompressive surgery for MMI reduces mortality and increases the number of patients with a favourable functional outcome.
- HAMLET: Surgical decompression within 48 h of onset of symptomatic MCA infarction did not improve functional outcomes compared to medical treatment.
- HeaDDFIRST: There was no difference in mortality at 180 days between surgical or medical management.

Critique

The pooled analysis of three ongoing trials is almost unique in the literature and the results of this pooled analysis are in keeping with reported findings from uncontrolled case series. However, one of the most fundamental dilemmas facing neurosurgeons is highlighted by the results of these studies and that is the question of what constitutes a 'favourable' outcome. An mRS ≤3 is generally accepted as 'favourable' but the pooled analysis used mRS ≤4, thereby including patients who were left with moderately severe disability. In fact, although surgery reduced mortality, a greater number of survivors (10-fold) are left with moderately severe disability. The authors of the pooled analysis have been careful to emphasize, therefore, that patients and clinicians need to be willing to accept the possibility of this survival outcome. From one perspective, therefore, hemicraniectomy for MMI is a life-saving procedure. An alternative view is that hemicraniectomy saves live at the cost of producing unacceptable levels of disability in the survivors. Indeed, the validity of trial designs that dichotomize outcomes into 'favourable' and 'unfavourable' has been widely criticized in the literature and it has been pointed out by numerous people that 'favourable' is not necessarily synonymous with 'acceptable' or 'desirable' outcomes.

Various criticisms have been raised against these trials, including the issue of whether of non-blinding of treatment arms had any effect on patient management, and in particular the use of intensive care resources in the two groups. For example, in the DECIMAL trial all patients undergoing surgery received mechanical ventilation, as compared to just over only two-thirds of patients managed medically. Whether this was an effect of non-blinding remains open to question (Mayer, 2007).

Various other concerns regarding the results and the way in which physicians and surgeons will use the information have been raised. For example, there is a tendency to avoid hemicraniectomy in patients with dominant hemisphere MMI due to the perception that global aphasia is a cruel outcome that should be avoided at all costs. Mayer has pointed out that the benefit of hemicraniectomy in the pooled analysis was independent of the presence or absence of aphasia and that dominant hemisphere involvement may not necessarily be an acceptable reason for withholding hemicraniectomy (Mayer, 2007).

One of the greatest criticisms of these trials is whether the criteria for patient selection can really reflect any degree of understanding of the natural history of malignant MCA infarction. The processes that determine which patients develop fatal brain oedema are not understood and there is clearly a need for larger imaging studies to evaluate the natural history of these lesions before we can fully elucidate the role of surgical or other interventions.

The decision to perform hemicraniectomy for MMI is still a matter for consideration on an individual case-by-case basis. Issues regarding the optimal timing of surgery still need to be resolved. The authors of the HAMLET trial updated the pooled analysis of the DESTINY/DECIMAL/HAMLET trials and reported a benefit of surgery for those operated on within 48 h of onset of stroke symptoms. However, no conclusions can be drawn about those patients operated on after this time period. Age is certainly an important factor with regard to outcome as it appears that the mortality even with surgery for patients over 50 with MMI is more than twice that of patients <50 (Gupta et al., 2005). Surgical decompression for MMI remains a complex dilemma for physicians, surgeons, and their patients.

Gupta R, Conolly ES, Mayer S, Elkind MS. Hemicraniectomy for massive middle cerebral artery territory infarction: a systematic review. *Stroke* 2004; **35**: 539–543.

Mayer SA. Hemicraniectomy: a second chance on life for patients with space-occupying MCA infarction. *Stroke* 2007; **38**: 2410–2412.

1.10 **Carotid endarterectomy for carotid stenosis**

Details of study

Carotid surgery for patients with symptomatic carotid stenosis has been performed for over 50 years but until 1991, no large, comprehensive trial had been conducted. The North American Symptomatic Carotid Endarterectomy Trial (NASCET) started recruiting in 1987 and initial reports were published in 1991. NASCET was a pivotal trial as it demonstrated that symptomatic patients with 70–99% stenosis benefited from surgery as compared to conservative management. Indeed, a clinical alert in 1991 stated that for 70–99% stenosis, surgery was clearly beneficial and recruitment of this group was stopped. Other trials in the 1990s include the European Carotid Surgery Trial (ECST) and the Veterans Affairs Cooperative Symptomatic Carotid Stenosis Trial. These were followed by the Asymptomatic Carotid Atherosclerosis Study (ACAS) in 1995 that suggested that asymptomatic patients with greater than 60% stenosis would benefit from surgery. More recently, with the advent of carotid stenting, trials have compared surgery to interventional radiological procedures. These are discussed in a separate section. In this section, we focus on the NASCET trial.

Study references

Main studies

Barnett HJ, Taylor DW, Eliasziw M, Fox AJ, Ferguson GG, Haynes RB, Rankin RN, Clagett GP, Hachinski VC, Sackett DL, Thorpe KE, Meldrum HE, Spence JD for the North American Symptomatic Carotid Endarterectomy Trial Collaborators. Benefit of carotid endarterectomy in patients with symptomatic moderate or severe stenosis. *N Engl J Med* 1998; **339**: 1415–1425.

The North American Symptomatic Carotid Endarterectomy Trial Collaborators. Beneficial effect of carotid endarterectomy in symptomatic patients with high-grade carotid stenosis. *N Engl J Med* 1991; **325**: 445–453.

National Institute of Neurological Disorders and Stroke, Stroke and Trauma Division. North American Symptomatic Carotid Endarterectomy Trial (NASCET) investigators. Clinical alert: benefit of carotid endarterectomy for patients with high-grade stenosis of the internal carotid artery. *Stroke* 1991; **22**: 816–817.

Related studies

European Carotid Surgery Trialists' Group. Randomized trial of endarterectomy for recently symptomatic carotid stenosis: final results of the MRC European Carotid Surgery Trial (ECST). *Lancet* 1998; **351**: 1379–1387.

Mayberg MR, Wilson SE, Yatsu F, Weiss DG, Messina L, Hershey LA, Colling C, Eskridge J, Deykin D, Winn HR. Veterans Affairs Cooperative Studies Program 309 Trialist Group. Carotid endarterectomy and prevention of cerebral ischaemia in symptomatic carotid stenosis. *JAMA* 1991; **266**: 3289–3294.

Executive Committee for the Asymptomatic Carotid Atherosclerosis Study. Endarterectomy for asymptomatic carotid artery stenosis. *JAMA* 1995; **273**: 1421–1428.

Paciaroni M, Eliasziw M, Sharpe BL, Kappelle J, Chaturvedi S, Meldrum H, Barnett HJM. Long-term clinical and angiographic outcomes in symptomatic patients with 70% to 90% carotid artery stenosis. *Stroke* 2000; **31**: 2037–2042.

Study design

• Non-blinded multi-centre RCT

Class of evidence	I
Randomization	Carotid endarterectomy versus medical management
Number of patients	659 (After 1991, 131, i.e. not 70–99% stenosis)
Follow-up	Mean = 3.6 years for medical group Mean = 7.0 years for surgical group
	Primary endpoint: Ipsilateral stroke
	Secondary endpoints: Any stroke Death
Number of centres	50
Stratification	By degree of stenosis i.e. <70% or 70–99%. A subsequent analysis divided the latter into 70–84% and 85–99%

• Patients were randomized within 120 days of diagnosis of severe carotid bifurcation stenosis and ipsilateral transient ischaemic attack or stroke.

• This was the first randomized study to show that surgery is beneficial for 70–99% stenosis.

• Multiplanar anteroposterior, oblique, and lateral selective ICA angiogram was required.

• Before 1991, 4-monthly clinic visits. After 1991, annual visits, bi-annual telephone assessments. If a stroke occurred, the patient had an extra clinic visit.

• All patients underwent annual carotid ultrasound scans.

• All patients had enteric-coated aspirin as well as antihypertensive, antilipidaemic, and antidiabetic therapies, if required.

• Several later studies including those in Europe showed similar results.

• Inclusion criteria: Transient ischaemic attack or disabling stroke plus severe carotid bifurcation stenosis within 120 days; age ≤80 years; consent.

• Exclusion criteria: Cardiac source of potential embolism; angiographic evidence of intracranial lesion > extracranial lesion; other life-threatening or disabling conditions.

Outcome Measures

Primary endpoint

• Fatal or non-fatal stroke ipsilateral to the randomized carotid artery

Secondary endpoints
- Strokes in any territory
- Death

Results

Baseline characteristics were similar in the two groups. In February 1991, an interim report (cited above) demonstrated that, in 659 patients with severe stenosis (70–99%), endarterectomy was associated with an absolute reduction of 17% in the risk of ipsilateral stroke at 2 years. Therefore, patients with severe stenosis were not enrolled after 1991 but were continued to be followed up until 1997. Enrolment of patients with <70% stenosis continued until 1996. The overall results showed that in the 50–69% stenosis group, the 5-year ipsilateral stroke rate was 15.7% in the surgical group compared to 22.2% in the medical group ($p = 0.045$). In the <50% stenosis group, there was no significant difference between surgical and medical treatments ($p = 0.16$). In the severe stenosis group (70–99%), the 30-day rate of disabling ipsilateral stroke or death was 2.1% and this increased to 6.7% at 8 years. Benefits were greatest for men, those with hemispheric symptoms, and recent stroke.

Conclusions

Patients with severe carotid bifurcation stenosis (70–99%) have a clear benefit from endarterectomy that is long lasting. Those with 50–69% have a moderate benefit, and other risk factors as well as surgeon skill should be taken into account. Surgery for stenosis <50% does not yield any benefit.

Critique

The results of the NASCET trial were further corroborated by the European Carotid Surgery Trial (ECST) that showed a 11.6% risk reduction of stroke at 3 years following surgery, in patients with >60% stenosis. Also similar to NASCET, the trial demonstrated that symptomatic patients with <40% stenosis had a worse outcome if treated surgically. The benefit of endarterectomy for asymptomatic patients is somewhat more controversial. The Asymptomatic Carotid Atherosclerosis Study (ACAS) demonstrated a significant 5.9% reduction in perioperative stroke or death and stroke at 5 years following surgery. However, in this trial, the investigators had an extremely low 30-day complication rate of only 2.3% (stroke or death). Similarly, the surgical complication rate was only 6% in the NASCET trial. These results imply that in order to get a 17% absolute reduction in stroke or death, a surgeon needs to have a complication rate of 6% or less. For the symptomatic, severe stenosis group, there is clear benefit from endarterectomy but in the moderate group, a surgeon has to be near the NASCET investigators rate or better to see a benefit.

Timing of surgery is an important factor. The cumulative risk results in this study show that the greatest risk of stroke is in the first 6 months of symptoms with a decrease continuing until approximately 2 years. After this, the difference between surgery and conservative treatment is less clear. Therefore, when interpreting the trial results, surgeons should consider whether the patients still have symptoms as well as the degree of stenosis.

Another important factor to consider is the how the degree of stenosis has been measured. In the NASCET trial, all patients underwent angiography. The trial investigators state that the narrowest portion of the stenosis should not be compared to the area of post-stenotic dilatation as this would yield false results. As the trial used angiography, it says nothing about the degree of stenosis as measured by ultrasonography, a technique commonly used by some centres. This question has been the subject of other subsequent studies and is beyond the scope of this section.

This large, randomized, multi-centre trial unequivocally demonstrated that surgery for 70–99% carotid stenosis reduces the rate of stroke or death and that this is a long-lasting effect. The publication of the 1991 Clinical Alert as well as the 1998 paper had a profound effect on the rates of carotid endarterectomy. Prior to this, rates of carotid endarterectomy fell as studies questioned the use of the procedure. After the NASCET trial, indications for surgery were clearly defined, and provided operations were performed by skilled surgeons in high-volume centres, benefit was clear. Therefore, rates increased in the 1990s but in selected patients. These results were subsequently confirmed.

1.11 **Carotid endarterectomy versus carotid stenting for carotid stenosis**

Details of study

Following the results of the NASCET trial (see Section 1.10), treatment protocols for patients with symptomatic, severe carotid stenosis became better defined. With the advancement of endovascular stenting techniques, it became inevitable that stenting of carotid arteries would become a viable alternative to surgery. But which technique is better and which has the lowest complication rate? There are a number of studies in the 10-year period from 1998 to 2008 that have looked at this. These include two large, multi-centre European trials (SPACE and EVA-3S) that recruited 1200 and 527 patients respectively, and CAVATAS that recruited 504 patients (Eckstein *et al.*, 2008; Mas *et al.*, 2008; Coward *et al.*, 2007). There have also been a number of smaller randomized trials including SAPPHIRE, WALLSTENT, Leicester, Kentucky A, and Kentucky B. Two other large multi-centre trials (ICSS and CREST) are ongoing. On the basis of these studies, there are only minor differences between treatments in the immediate (30-day) period after surgery but longer-term follow-up may show differences. Here we concentrate on the SPACE study as it is the largest and one of the earlier trials.

Study references

Main study

Eckstein HH, Ringleb P, Allenberg JR, Berger J, Fraedrich G, Hacke W, Hennerici M, Stingele R, Fiehler J, Zeumer H, Jansen O. Results of the Stent-Protected Angioplasty versus Carotid Endarterectomy (SPACE) study to treat symptomatic stenoses at 2 years: a multinational, prospective, randomised trial. *Lancet Neurol* 2008; **7**: 893–902.

Related studies

Mas JL, Trinquart L, Leys D, Albucher JF, Rousseau H, Viguier A, Bossavy JP, Denis B, Piquet P, Garnier P, Viader F, Touzé E, Julia P, Giroud M, Krause D, Hosseini H, Becquemin JP, Hinzelin G, Houdart E, Hénon H, Neau JP, Bracard S, Onnient Y, Padovani R, Chatellier G; EVA-3S investigators. Endarterectomy Versus Angioplasty in Patients with Symptomatic Severe Carotid Stenosis (EVA-3S) trial: results up to 4 years from a randomised, multicentre trial. *Lancet Neurol* 2008; **7**: 885–892.

Coward LJ, McCabe DJ, Ederle J, Featherstone RL, Clifton A, Brown MM; CAVATAS Investigators. Long-term outcome after angioplasty and stenting for symptomatic vertebral artery stenosis compared with medical treatment in the Carotid And Vertebral Artery Transluminal Angioplasty Study (CAVATAS): a randomized trial. *Stroke* 2007; **38**: 1526–1530.

Gurm HS, Yadav JS, Fayad P, Katzen BT, Mishkel GJ, Bajwa TK, Ansel G, Strickman NE, Wang H, Cohen SA, Massaro JM, Cutlip DE; SAPPHIRE Investigators. Long-term results of carotid stenting versus endarterectomy in high-risk patients. *N Engl J Med* 2008; **358**: 1572–1579.

Study design

- PRCT

Class of evidence	I
Randomization	Non-blinded carotid endarterectomy versus carotid stenting
Number of patients	613 assigned to stenting versus 601 assigned to surgery
Length of follow-up	2 years
Number of centres	36
Stratification	All patients have at least 70% stenosis according to ECST or 50% according to NASCET

- SPACE is one of the largest early trials looking at stent versus surgery for carotid stenosis.
- It is the equivalent of NASCET except that the two conditions are surgery and stenting rather than surgery and conservative treatment.
- Essentially, the study showed that there is little difference in outcome between the two groups. However, the degree of re-stenosis is higher in the stent group.
- The results of this study are similar to other stent versus surgery trials.
- Each centre had to demonstrate, in advance, their expertise in dealing with carotid artery stenosis, and quality committees were set up to define guidelines. Multidisciplinary teams comprising interventionalists, vascular surgeons, and neurologists decided on each case.
- Inclusion criteria: Symptomatic stenosis (transient ischaemic attack (TIA) or stroke) of carotid bifurcation or internal carotid artery within 180 days (proven by Duplex sonography or angiography); modified Rankin score 2 or less; > 50 years of age; informed consent.
- Exclusion criteria: Intracranial haemorrhage within last 90 days; uncontrolled arterial hypertension; known intracranial angioma; < 2 years life expectancy; aspirin, clopidogrel, or ASS contraindicated; contrast media contraindicated; planned simultaneous surgery; stenosis due to other reasons— external compression, dissection, recurrent after surgery, fibromuscular dysplasia, floating thrombus, intracranial stenosis, and 100% stenosis.

Outcome measures

Primary endpoints

- Ipsilateral stroke (cerebral infarction and/or bleeding with longer than 24 h functional impairment) or death (any cause) from randomization up to 30th day (± 3 days) from treatment

Secondary endpoints

◆ Ipsilateral stroke or death from vascular causes within 24 months ± 14 days from randomization

◆ Re-stenosis of at least 70% on Duplex sonography at 6, 12, 24 months ± 14 days from randomization

◆ Procedural technical failure, including re-stenosis on 6th ± 1 day or 30th ± 3 days from treatment

◆ Ipsilateral stroke with Rankin score of 3 or more from randomization up to 30 ± 3 days

◆ Incidence of any strokes within 30 ± 3 days

◆ Incidence of any strokes within 24 months ± 14 days

Results

There were no differences in baseline characteristics between the two groups; 601 were randomized to endarterectomy and 613 to stenting. The 30-day rates of primary endpoint events in the intention-to-treat analysis was 6.45% in the surgery group versus 6.92% in the angioplasty group ($p = 0.09$). With adjustment for major protocol violations, this was 5.51% in the surgery versus 6.81% in the angioplasty group. Indeed, carotid endarterectomy patients tended to have better outcomes in most of the 30-day endpoints. More patients in the angioplasty group received double antiplatelet treatment (e.g. aspirin and clopidogrel) than in the surgery group. With regard to 2-year outcomes, there were no significant differences but the trend was for fewer complications in the surgery group. With regard to mortality, there were 32 deaths in the angioplasty group, compared to 28 in the carotid endarterectomy group (Kaplan–Meier estimates of 6.2% and 4.9% respectively ($p = 0.63$). The Kaplan–Meier estimates of ipsilateral strokes or death within 2 years plus any periprocedural strokes or death was 9.5% in the stenting group versus 8.8% in the surgery group ($p = 0.62$). Recurrent stenosis of 70% or more was significantly more common in the stenting group (10.7%) compared to the surgery group (4.6%, $p = 0.0009$).

Subgroup analyses revealed that there was an age-related increase in primary outcome events in patients with carotid angioplasty with stenting compared to no change across age groups in the surgical group. This means that patients less than 68 years of age had a lower periprocedural risk in the angioplasty group and carotid endarterectomy had a lower periprocedural risk in those patients over 68 years.

Conclusions

This study failed to show a non-inferiority of carotid angioplasty and stenting versus carotid endarterectomy for the 30-day complication rates. Indeed, overall, surgery was the favourable option. However, there was no difference between the two treatments and risk of cerebrovascular events at 2 years.

Critique

The SPACE trial is a large, randomized trial that failed to show that carotid artery stenting is better than carotid endarterectomy. However, as commented on by Wiesmann *et al.* (2008), the trial was based on a frequency of 5% to reach the primary endpoint in each treatment arm. As the frequency was much higher in each arm, it was underpowered to establish non-inferiority of stenting versus surgery and would require a further 1200 to 1800 patients. However, the results agree broadly with most of the other similar trials that are listed above. The main difference with the SAPPHIRE trial is that the latter looks at patients at high risk for carotid endarterectomy and as a consequence has higher complication rates for both treatments. One of the main criticisms of these trials is that the follow-up (usually limited to 2 years) is aimed at complications related to the procedures rather than long-term re-stenosis rates. If long-term re-stenosis is due to progression of atherosclerosis, one might expect re-stenosis to take longer than 2 years. There is some evidence that most of the re-stenoses in the trial were related to intimal hyperplasia and this may have overestimated the incidence, though this has not been proven. A further criticism, stated by the SPACE investigators themselves, is that the trial did not look at secondary prevention strategies such as lipid-lowering drugs or smoking status.

In summary of all of the studies, carotid angioplasty plus stenting has been shown to have slightly higher periprocedural (up to 30 days) stroke risk but surgery has a higher rate of cranial nerve palsy or myocardial infarction. There is no difference between the periprocedural disabling stroke and death risks between the two groups. Also, there is no evidence that an embolic protection device influences outcome. Therefore, surgery is still the standard treatment for this condition but two further trials—ICSS and CREST, with large patient numbers, are awaited.

Impact on field

This study has shown that there is little advantage of stenting over surgery for carotid stenosis, but at the same time there are only minor differences in complication rates. The main question now is whether the long-term re-stenosis rates will be any different and this will necessitate the outcomes of the CREST and ICSS trials.

Wiesmann M, Schöpf V, Jansen O, Brückmann H. Stent-protected angioplasty versus carotid endarterectomy in patients with carotid artery stenosis: meta-analysis of randomized trial data. *Eur Radiol* 2008 Jul 25 (epub ahead of print).

Chapter 2

Neuro-oncology

RD Johnson, KJ Drummond, KJOL Khu, M Bernstein

2.0 **Introduction**

Controversies and debate in neuro-oncology are relevant to the practice of every neurosurgeon. There is a wealth of published literature in this area that continues to expand, seemingly exponentially. We have included, therefore, in this chapter a selection of studies that address certain key issues that we feel are directly relevant to the practising neuro-oncological surgeon today.

We open this chapter by considering a randomized trial of the role of steroids in the management of cerebral oedema associated with brain tumours. The use of dexamethasone for this purpose was the result of work by Joseph Galicich, Lyle French, and James Melby from the University of Minnesota in the 1960s (Galicich *et al.*, 1961). Their work has been described as 'one of the greatest contributions in the history of neurosurgery' and we would recommend that the interested reader consult a recent legacy review of the original work by McLelland and Long (McLelland and Long, 2008). The study chosen for inclusion in this chapter is the randomized trial carried out by Vecht *et al.* in the Netherlands to establish the efficacy and optimal dosing regime for dexamethasone (Vecht *et al.*, 1994).

The next two sections address two important areas of neuro-oncology: the role of surgery and adjuvant radiotherapy for single brain metastases. Brain metastases occur in approximately 25% of patients with cancer and constitute the most common type of brain tumour. In those patients without a known primary lesion, neurosurgical intervention may be necessary in order to obtain a tissue diagnosis. In those with multiple cerebral metastases, radiotherapy is the accepted treatment option. However, the situation is more complex in patients with a single brain metastasis and known extracranial disease and we have included the three largest and most widely referenced trials that have addressed the role of surgery in addition to radiotherapy in this situation (Patchell *et al.*, 1990; Vecht *et al.*, 1993; Mintz *et al.*, 1996). We have also included the only randomized trial to consider the role of radiotherapy as an adjunct to surgery for a single brain metastasis (Patchell *et al.*, 1998). There is considerable controversy regarding the role of surgery for multiple cerebral metastases, and a survey of the literature reveals several conflicting views from published case series. Perhaps in a future edition we will be able to critique the results of a randomized controlled trial in this area. Stereotactic radiosurgery for brain metastases has also been evaluated by two prospective randomized trials and we have included these here (Andrews *et al.*, 2004; Aoyama *et al.*, 2006).

The next sections of the chapter deal with the management of high-grade gliomas. Numerous studies have attempted to address the role of surgical resection in malignant gliomas and particularly whether 'total' resection is really beneficial. We have included three of the larger and well-designed studies addressing this issue (Keles *et al.*, 1999; Vuorinen *et al.*, 2003; Stummer *et al.*, 2006). Following on from this we have looked at key studies evaluating the role of chemotherapy in high-grade glioma. The benefits of chemotherapy in glioblastoma have been controversial and this has been reflected by different approaches to the treatment of glioblastoma in Europe and the United States over the last 25 years. The role of early concomitant systemic temozolomide chemotherapy for glioblastoma was evaluated by the European Organisation for Research and Treatment of Cancer Brain Tumour and Radiotherapy Groups (EORTC) and the National Cancer Institute of Canada Clinical Trials Group (NCIC) and is familiarly known as the 'temozolomide trial' (Stupp *et al.*, 2005). This trial showed the greatest improvement in mortality since the Brain Tumour Study Group established the benefits of radiotherapy in 1978 (Walker *et al.*, 1978). This temozolomide trial has led to the routine use of temozolomide chemotherapy in patients with glioblastomas. There is also a growing body of evidence to support the role of localized chemotherapy by way of carmustine wafers and we have included the two largest trials conducted on this issue (Brem *et al.*, 1995; Valtonen *et al.*, 1997; Westphal *et al.*, 2003, 2006).

The next section considers brachytherapy for high-grade gliomas. This modality received quite a bit of attention in the 1980s. Several large randomized controlled trials, however, found that it was of no benefit. These are landmark studies as the findings resulted in the discontinuation of this therapy. We have considered two of these landmark trials in this section (Laperriere *et al.*, 1998; Selker *et al.*, 2002).

The last two sections deal with low-grade gliomas. The penultimate section considers two retrospective studies which evaluate the extent of resection on outcome for low-grade gliomas (McGirt *et al.*, 2008; Smith *et al.*, 2008). The role of radiotherapy in the management low-grade gliomas presents a difficult dilemma for the neurosurgical oncologist. Several trials have been carried out to address this issue: EORTC I ('believers trial'); EORTC II ('non-believers trial'); and NCCTG-RTOG-ECOG trial ('US trial'). We have, therefore, included a final section that looks at these trials together (Karim *et al.*, 1996; Karim *et al.*, 2002; Shaw *et al.*, 2002; van den Bent *et al.*, 2005).

Andrews DW, Scott CB, Sperduto PW, Flanders AE, Gaspar LE, Schell MC, Werner-Wasik M, Demas W, Ryu J, Bahary JP, Souhami L, Rotman M, Mehta MP, Curran WJ Jr. Whole brain radiation therapy with or without stereotactic radiosurgery boost for patients with one to three brain metastases: phase III results of the RTOG 9508 randomised trial. *Lancet* 2004; **363**: 1655–1672.

Aoyama H, Shirato H, Tago T, Nakagawa K, Toyoda T, Hatano K, Kenjyo M, Oya N, Hirota S, Shioura H, Kunieda E, Inomata T, Hayakawa K, Katoh N, Kobashi G. Stereotactic radiosurgery plus whole-brain radiation therapy vs stereotactic radiosurgery alone for the treatment of brain metastases – a randomised controlled trial. *JAMA* 2006; **21**: 2483–2491.

Brem H, Piantadosi S, Burger PC, Walker M, Selker R, Vick NA, Black K, Sisti M, Brem S, Mohr G, Muller P, Morawetz R, Schold SC, for the Polymer-Brain Tumor Treatment Group. Placebo-controlled trial of safety and efficacy of intraoperative controlled delivery by biodegradable polymers of chemotherapy for recurrent gliomas. *Lancet* 1995; **345**: 1008–1012.

Galicich JH, French LA, Melby JC. Use of dexamethasone in treatment of cerebral oedema associated with brain tumours. *Lancet* 1961; **81**: 46–53.

Karim AB, Maat B, Hatlevoll R, Menten J, Rutten EH, Thomas DG, Mascarenhas F, Horiot JC, Parvinen LM, van Reijn M, Jager JJ, Fabrini MG, van Alphen AM, Hamers HP, Gaspar L, Noordman E, Pierart M, van Glabbeke M. A randomized trial on dose-response in radiation therapy of low-grade cerebral glioma. European Organization for Research and Treatment of Cancer (EORTC) Study 22844. *Int J Rad Oncol Biol Phys* 1996; **36**: 549–556.

Karim AB, Afra D, Cornu P, Bleehen N, Schraub S, De Witte O, Darcel F, Stenning S, Pierart M, Van Glabbeke M. Randomised trial on the efficacy of radiotherapy for cerebral low-grade glioma in the adult: European Organization for Research and Treatment of Cancer Study 22844 with the Medical Research Council study BRO4: an interim analysis. *Int J Rad Oncol Biol Phys* 2002; **52**: 316–324.

Keles GE, Anderson B, Berger MS. The effect of extent of resection on time to tumor progression and survival in patients with glioblastoma mulitforme of the cerebral hemisphere. *Cancer* 1999; **74**: 1784–1791.

Laperriere NJ, Leung PM, McKenzie S, Milosevic M, Wong S, Glen J, Pintilie M, Bernstein M. Randomized study of brachytherapy in the initial management of patients with malignant astrocytoma. *Int J Radiat Oncol Biol Phys* 1998; **41**: 1005–1011.

McGirt MJ, Chaichana KL, Attenello FJ, Weingart JD, Than K, Burger PC, Olivi A, Brem H, Quinones-Hinojosa A. Extent of surgical resection is independently associated with survival in patients with hemispheric infiltrating low-grade gliomas. *Neurosurgery* 2008; **63**: 700–708.

McLelland S, Long DM. Genesis of the use of corticosteroids in the treatment and prevention of brain oedema. *Neurosurgery* 2008; **62**: 965–968.

Mintz AH, Kestle J, Rathbone MP, Gaspar L, Hugenholtz H, Fisher B, Duncan G, Skingley P, Foster G, Levine M. A randomized trial to assess the efficacy of surgery in addition to radiotherapy in patients with a single cerebral metastasis. *Cancer* 1996; **78**: 1470–1476.

Patchell RA, Tibbs PA, Walsh JW, Dempsey RJ, Maruyama Y, Kryscio RJ, Markesbery WR, Macdonald JS, Young B. A randomized trial of surgery in the treatment of single metastases to the brain. *N Eng J Med* 1990; **322**: 494–500.

Patchell RA, Tibbs PA, Regine WF, Dempsey RJ, Mohiuddin M, Kryscio RJ, Markesbery WR, Foon KA, Young B. Postoperative radiotherapy in the treatment of single metastases to the brain: a randomized trial. *JAMA* 1998; **280**: 1485–1489.

Selker RG, Shapiro WR, Burger P, Blackwood MS, Deutsch M, Arena VA, Van Gilder JC, Wu J, Malkin MG, Mealey J, Neal JH, Olson J, Robertson JT, Barnett GH, Bloomfield S, Albright R, Hochberg FH, Hiesiger E, Green S. The Brain Tumor Cooperative Group NIH Trial 87–01: A randomized comparison of surgery, external radiotherapy, and carmustine versus surgery, interstitial radiotherapy boost, external radiation therapy, and carmustine. *Neurosurgery* 2002; **51**: 343–357.

Shaw E, Arusell R, Scheithauer B, O'Fallon J, O'Neill B, Dinapoli R, Nelson D, Earle J, Jones C, Cascino T, Nichols D, Ivnik R, Hellman R, Curran W, Abrams R. Prospective randomized trial of low- versus high-dose radiation therapy in adults with supratentorial low-grade glioma: initial report of a North Central Cancer Treatment Group/Radiation Therapy Oncology Group/Eastern Cooperative Oncology Group Study. *J Clin Oncol* 2002; **20**: 2267–2276.

Smith JS, Chang EF, Lamborn KR, Chang SM, Prados MD, Cha S, Tihan T, Vandenberg S. Role of extent of resection in the long-term outcome of low-grade hemispheric gliomas. *J Clin Oncol* 2008; **10**: 1338–1345.

Stummer W, Pichlmeier U, Meinel T, Wiestler OD, Zanella F, Reulen HJ; ALA-Glioma Study Group. Fluorescence-guided surgery with 5-aminolevulinic acid for resection of malignant glioma: a randomised controlled mulitcentre phase III trial. *Lancet Oncol* 2006; **7**: 392–401.

Stupp R, Mason WP, van den Bent MJ, Weller M, Fisher B, Taphoorn MJB, Belander K, Brande AA, Marosi C, Bogdahn U, Curschmann K, Janzer RC, Ludwin SK, Gorlia T, Allgeier A, Lacombe D, Cairncross G, Eisenhauer E, Mirimanoff RO, for the European Organisation for Research and Treatment of Cancer Brain Tumour and Radiotherapy Groups and the National Cancer Institute of Canada Clinical Trials Group. Radiotherapy plus concomitant and adjuvant temozolomide for glioblastoma. *N Engl J Med* 2005; **352**: 987–996.

Valtonen S, Timonen U, Toivanen P, Kalimo H, Kivipetto L, Heiskanen O, Unsgaard G, Kuurne T. Interstitial chemotherapy with carmustine with carmustine-loaded polymers for high-grade gliomas: a randomised double-blind study. *Neurosurgery* 1997; **41**: 44–48.

Van den Bent MJ, Afra D, de Witte O, Ben Hassel M, Schraub S, Hoang-Xuan K, Malmström PO, Collette L, Piérart M, Mirimanoff R, Karim AB. EORTC Radiotherapy and Brain Tumor Groups and the UK Medical Research Council. Long-term efficacy of early versus delayed radiotherapy for low-grade astrocytoma and oligodendroglioma in adults: the EORTC 22845 randomised trial. *Lancet* 2005; **366**: 985–990.

Vecht CJ, Haaxma-Reiche H, Noordijk EM, Padberg GW, Voormenolen JH, Hoekstra FM, Tans JT, Lambooij N, Metsaars JA, Wattendorf AR, Brand R, Hermans J. Treatment of single brain metastasis: radiotherapy alone or combined with neurosurgery? *Ann Neurol* 1993; **33**: 583–590.

Vecht CJ, Hovestadt A, Verbiest HB, Verbiest HB, van Vliet JJ, van Putten WL. Dose-effect relationship of dexamethasone on Karnofsky performance in metastatic brain tumors: a randomized controlled study of doses 4, 8 and 16 mg per day. *Neurology* 1994; **44**: 675–680.

Vuorinen V, Hinkka S, Farkilla M, Jasskelainen J. Debulking or biopsy of malignant glioma in elderly people – a randomized study. *Acta Neurochir (Wein)* 2003; **145**: 5–10.

Walker MD, Alexanderander E Jr, Hunt WE, MacCarty CS, Mahaley MS Jr, Mealey J Jr, Norrell HA, Owens G, Ransohoff J, Wilson CB, Gehan EA, Strike TA. Evaluation of BCNU and/or radiotherapy in the treatment of anaplastic gliomas. A cooperative clinical trial. *J Neurosurg* 1978; **49**: 333–343.

Westphal M, Hilt DC, Bortey E, Delavault P, Olivares R, Wamke PC, Whittle IR, Jääskeäinen J, Ram Z. A phase 3 trial of local chemotherapy with biodegradable carmustine (BCNU) wafers (Gliadel wafers) in patients with primary malignant glioma. *Neuro-Oncology* 2003; **5**: 79–88.

Westphal M, Ram Z, Riddle V, Hilt D, Bortey E. Gliadel wafer in initial surgery for malignant glioma: long-term follow-up of a multi-center controlled trial. *Acta Neurochir (Wein)* 2006; **148**: 269–275.

2.1 Steroids for the management of cerebral oedema associated with brain tumours

Details of study

This is the only randomized study addressing the therapeutic efficacy of steroids to manage cerebral oedema in patients with brain tumours. The trial was carried out in the Netherlands in the early 1990s.

Study references

Main study

Vecht CJ, Hovestadt A, Verbiest HB, Verbiest HB, van Vliet JJ, van Putten WL. Dose-effect relationship of dexamethasone on Karnofsky performance in metastatic brain tumors: a randomized controlled study of doses 4, 8 and 16 mg per day. *Neurology* 1994; **44**: 675–680.

Related reference

Galicich JH, French LA, Melby JC. Use of dexamethasone in treatment of cerebral oedema associated with brain tumours. *J Lancet* 1961; **81**: 46–53.

Study design

♦ Double-blind randomized controlled trial (RCT)

Class of evidence	I
Randomization	Low-dose versus high-dose dexamethasone
Number of patients	96
Follow-up	8 weeks
	Primary endpoints: Neurological status Functional status Quality of life
	Secondary endpoints: Side effects
Number of centres	1
Stratification	None

♦ Included patients: Metastatic brain tumours on computed tomography (CT); Karnofsky score ≤80.

♦ Patients randomized between 4, 8, and 16 mg/day of dexamethasone but in two series: Series 1 (8 mg versus 16 mg); Series 2 (4 mg versus 16 mg).

Outcome measures

Primary endpoints

- Neurological status
- Functional status (Karnofsky score)
- Quality of life
- Side effects: Standardized questionnaire and clinical examination
- Assessment at 1, 4, and 8 weeks

Results

Outcome		Series 1			Series 2		
		8 mg	16 mg	Statistical significance	4 mg	16 mg	Statistical significance
Improvement in Karnofsky score	1 week	60%	54%	None	67%	70%	None
	4 weeks	53%	81%	None	62%	60%	None

- Ninety-two percent follow-up at 4 weeks.
- Although patients receiving 16 mg/day had approximately 25% improvement on proximal muscle weakness in the first month there was no significant improvement in the subsequent month.
- Patients receiving 4 mg/day experienced <50% the number of Cushingoid faces as those receiving 16 mg/day ($p = 0.03$).
- There were no significant differences in the improvement of Karnofsky scores between dosing regimes at 1 week or any other time point.

Conclusions

- After 1 week, 4 mg is as effective as 16 mg of dexamethasone in patients with no impending signs of brain herniation.
- Toxic effects of dexamethasone are dose dependent and are much more frequent if 16 mg is administered for prolonged periods (1 month or more).

Critique

Brain oedema is one of the greatest factors contributing to neurological decline and impairment of quality of life in patients with brain tumours. The use of steroids in the management of brain tumours was established in the 1950s and 1960s after a number of observations by several clinicians. In 1957, Kofman et al. had noted the relief of neurological symptoms in a patient with metastatic breast cancer who received prednisolone for adrenal suppression (Kofman et al., 1957). They reported benefits from the administration of prednisolone to a series of 20 patients with brain tumours (Kofman *et al.*, 1957). Following this, Joseph Galicich, at the University of Minnesota, noted a circadian periodicity in the permeability of the blood–brain barrier in mice that was the directly reciprocal to the endogenous corticosteroid circadian rhythms. This observation led to a trial showing that dexamethasone was beneficial in treating in patients with neurological deficits from brain tumours (Galicich *et al.*, 1961). This study by Galicich *et al.* led to the widespread use of dexamethasone in the treatment of cerebral oedema associated with brain tumours and has been referred to as arguably the 'greatest translational research contribution in the history of neurosurgery' (McLelland and Long, 2008). The use of dexamethasone is associated with the risk of adverse effects including Cushingoid faces, psychosis, diabetes, and peptic ulceration. The later trial by Vecht *et al.* addresses the question of how the dose of dexamethasone affects efficacy and incidence of side effects. The follow-up period and outcome assessments used by Vecht and colleagues were appropriate to answer these questions. The trial design included two series because interim analysis revealed that the effect of a dose difference of 8 mg may be too small. The trial established the efficacy and dosing of dexamethasone for cerebral oedema in patients with brain tumours. Prior to this trial the standard dose of dexamethasone was 16 mg/day. On the basis of their results, Vecht and colleagues recommended the following dosing regimes:

Neurological status of patient	Dosing regimen
↓GCS or signs of ↑ICP/impending herniation	10 mg IV stat + 4 x 4 mg/day orally
GCS 15/15 + no signs of ↑ICP	4 mg/day orally

Galicich JH, French LA, Melby JC. Use of dexamethasone in treatment of cerebral oedema associated with brain tumours. *J Lancet* 1961; **81**: 46–53.

Kofman S, Garvin JS, Nagamani D, Taylor SG. Treatment of cerebral metastases from breast carcinoma with prednisolone. *JAMA* 1957; **163**: 1473–1476.

McLelland S, Long DM. Genesis of the use of corticosteroids in the treatment and prevention of brain oedema. *Neurosurgery* 2008; **62**: 965–968.

2.2 Surgery for single brain metastases

Details of studies

There have been three randomized trials evaluating the role of surgical resection in the treatment of solitary brain metastasis. All three trials compared surgical resection plus radiotherapy versus radiotherapy alone. The first study was carried out in the University of Kentucky in the United States between 1985 and 1989 (Patchell *et al.*, 1990). The second study was carried out in the Netherlands between 1985 and 1991 (Vecht *et al.*, 1993) and the third study was carried out in Canada (Mintz *et al.*, 1996).

Study references

Main studies

Patchell RA, Tibbs PA, Walsh JW, Dempsey RJ, Maruyama Y, Kryscio RJ, Markesbery WR, Macdonald JS, Young B. A randomized trial of surgery in the treatment of single metastases to the brain. *N Eng J Med* 1990; **322**: 494–500.

Vecht CJ, Haaxma-Reiche H, Noordijk EM, Padberg GW, Voormenolen JH, Hoekstra FH, Tans JT, Lambooij N, Metsaars JA, Wattendorf AR, Brand R, Hermans J. Treatment of single brain metastasis: radiotherapy alone or combined with neurosurgery? *Ann Neurol* 1993; **33**: 583–590.

Mintz AH, Kestle J, Rathbone MP, Gaspar L, Hugenholtz H, Fisher B, Duncan G, Skingley P, Foster G, Levine M. A randomized trial to assess the efficacy of surgery in addition to radiotherapy in patients with a single cerebral metastasis. *Cancer* 1996; **78**: 1470–1476.

Related references

Gaspar L, Scott C, Ratman M, Asbell S, Phillips T, Wasserman T, McKenna WG, Byhardt R. Recursive partitioning analysis (RPA) of prognostic factors in three radiation therapy oncology group (RTOG) brain metastases trials. *In J Radiat Oncol Biol Phys* 1997; **37**: 745–751.

Patchell RA, Tibbs PA, Regine WF, Dempsey RJ, Mohiuddin M, Kryscio RJ, Markesbery WR, Foon KA, Young B. Postoperative radiotherapy in the treatment of single metastases to the brain: a randomized trial. *JAMA* 1998; **280**: 1485–1489.

Study designs

- ◆ All RCTs

	Patchell *et al.* (1990)	Vecht *et al.* (1993)	Mintz *et al.* (1996)
Class of evidence	I	I	I
Randomization	Surgery + DXT versus DXT alone	Surgery + DXT versus DXT alone	Surgery + DXT versus DXT alone
Number of patients	48	63	84
Follow-up	100%	100%	100%
	Primary endpoints: Recurrence of brain metastasis Survival	Primary endpoint: Survival	Primary endpoint: Survival
	Secondary endpoints: Functional independent survival (FIS) Recurrence	Secondary endpoint: Functional independent survival (FIS)	Secondary endpoints: Functional status Quality of life

	Patchell et al. (1990)	Vecht et al. (1993)	Mintz et al. (1996)
Number of centres	1	5	7
Stratification	◆ Site of primary tumour ◆ Type of primary tumour ◆ Extent of extracranial activity of tumour	◆ Site of primary tumour ◆ Extent of extracranial activity of tumour	◆ Extent of extracranial activity of tumour ◆ Type of cancer (lung versus others) ◆ Size of metastasis (<3 cm versus ≥3 cm)

- Goals of surgery in all the three trials were total removal of the brain metastasis.
- Biopsy was undertaken to confirm the diagnosis in the radiotherapy arms in the studies by Patchell *et al.* and Mintz *et al.*, but not in the study by Vecht *et al.*
- Stratification by location consisted of dividing lesions into supratentorial and infratentorial groups.
- All trials carried out an intention-to-treat analysis.

Inclusion and exclusion criteria

	Patchell et al. (1990)	Vecht et al. (1993)	Mintz et al. (1996)
Inclusion criteria	◆ Age ≥18 ◆ Radiological confirmation of single brain metastasis ◆ Histological confirmation of systemic cancer within last 5 years ◆ Karnofsky Performance Score (KPS) ≥70	◆ Age ≥18 ◆ Histological confirmation of extracranial primary ◆ Radiological confirmation of single brain metastasis ◆ Good quality of life and neurological function ◆ Life expectancy of >6 months from extracranial disease	◆ Age <80 ◆ Radiological confirmation of single brain metastasis ◆ Pathologic confirmation of cancer within last 5 years (if not then biopsy performed to confirm) ◆ KPS >50
Exclusion criteria	◆ Brain lesions deemed unresectable ◆ Leptomeningeal disease ◆ Previous cranial radiotherapy ◆ Acute neurological deterioration requiring emergency surgery ◆ Certain tumours: Small cell lung CA; lymphoma; multiple myeloma; germ-cell tumours; leukaemia	◆ Small cell lung CA ◆ Malignant lymphoma ◆ Leptomeningeal/other intracranial deposits	◆ KPS <50 ◆ Leukaemia, lymphoma, small cell lung CA, non-melanomatous skin CA ◆ Previous cranial irradiation ◆ Meningeal carcinomatosis ◆ Previous cranial irradiation ◆ Brainstem or basal ganglia lesion ◆ Previous brain metastases ◆ Medical condition/co-morbidities preventing adequate follow-up

Outcome measures

Primary outcomes

- Survival was the primary outcome in all three trials.
- In addition, the recurrence of intracerebral metastasis was a primary outcome in the Patchell trial.

Secondary outcomes

Patchell et al. (1990)	• Recurrence at the site of the original metastasis was confirmed with CT or MRI scan • Quality of life defined as KPS of ≥70 (self-caring, but unable to work or maintain normal activity)
Vecht et al. (1993)	• Functional independent survival (FIS) defined as ≤1 on the 5-point WHO performance scale (0 = independent; 1 = symptoms but almost completely independent) and ≤1 on a 4-point neurological scale (0 = normal; 1 = minor symptoms)
Mintz et al. (1996)	• Functional status: Independence defined as proportion of time that patient had KPS of ≥70 • Quality of life: Measured using the Spitzer QOL 5-domain index

Results

- Follow-up for primary outcome was 100% in all the three trials.

Median survival

	Study								
	Patchell et al. (1990)			**Vecht et al. (1993)**			**Mintz et al. (1996)**		
Treatment	Surgery + WBRT	WBRT alone	Statistical significance	Surgery + WBRT	WBRT alone	Statistical significance	Surgery + WBRT	WBRT alone	Statistical significance
Median survival	40 weeks	15 weeks	$p < 0.01$	10 months	6 months	$p = 0.04$	5.6 months	6.3 months	None

Other significant findings

Patchell et al. (1990)

- With death from neurological causes used as an endpoint, median survival was greater in the surgery group compared to the whole brain radiotherapy (WBRT) group (62 weeks versus 26 weeks, $p < 0.0009$).
- Rate of recurrence of the original metastasis was much lower in the surgically treated group compared those treated with radiotherapy alone and that this was statistically significant (20% versus 52%, $p < 0.02$).

- Median length of time to recurrence was much lower in the surgery group compared to the WBRT group and this was statistically significant (21 weeks versus 59 weeks, $p < 0.0001$).
- Patients maintained quality of life (KPS ≥70) for much longer in the surgery group compared to the WBRT group and this was statistically significant (38 weeks versus 8 weeks, $p < 0.005$).

Vecht *et al.* (1993)

- Patients with stable extracranial disease had a better functional independent survival (FIS) with combined treatment ($p = 0.01$).

Mintz *et al.* (1996)

- There were no differences in the functional status or quality of life of patients in either treatment arm.

Conclusions

Two out of the three trials found that surgery plus radiotherapy is superior to radiotherapy alone for single cerebral metastasis.

- Patchell *et al.* concluded that surgery plus WBRT results in longer life, fewer recurrences of brain metastasis, and a better quality of life for patients with brain metastases.
- Vecht *et al.* concluded that surgery is beneficial for patients with single brain metastases and stable extracranial disease but WBRT is sufficient for patients with progressive extracranial disease within the previous 3 months.
- Mintz *et al.* concluded that the addition of surgery to radiation therapy did not improve the outcome of patients with a single brain metastasis.

Critique

Prior to 1990 the only evidence supporting the role of surgery for single cerebral metastases in patients with known systemic disease came from published case series that may have been biased by selecting only patients in good clinical condition for surgery. Uncontrolled case series looking at the effectiveness of surgery in brain metastases provided conflicting results and, therefore, the role of surgery in these patients remained to be determined. Previous studies had revealed that the median survival for untreated brain metastases is approximately 1 month but this could be improved to 3 months in the majority of patients with steroids and WBRT (Cairncross *et al.*, 1980). It is important to note that only half of patients with brain metastases have single metastasis. Of these, another half will not be eligible for surgery for reasons of extracranial disease. Therefore, only a small portion of patients with solitary brain metastasis are really candidates for surgery.

Patchell *et al.* analysed deaths according to whether they were from neurologic dysfunction or due to systemic disease. They found that the reason for the overall longer survival in the surgery group was a large reduction in deaths from neurological dysfunction, there being no effect on deaths from systemic disease. Overall survival was still <10% at 3 months in the Patchell *et al.* study. Thus, although no difference in long-term survival their results clearly favour a benefit of surgery in terms of survival and quality of life in patients with single metastases and limited, well-controlled extracranial disease. Patchell *et al.* found that the only two factors reducing the risk of recurrence of the original metastasis were surgical treatment and the absence of disseminated disease (multivariate analysis). However, surgery had no effect on the development of other brain metastases. In terms of quality of life they reported a significant benefit of surgery. However, older patients and those with disseminated disease were associated with poor quality of life.

A potential weakness of Patchell's 1990 study is that it is a small study and could, therefore, be affected by inadequate randomization and it reduces the probability of including long-term survivors of surgery (Posner, 1990). Nonetheless, their study represents a landmark in neurosurgery for being the first published RCT evaluating the role of surgery in the management of single brain metastases. Indeed, all three trials considered here are relatively small in size.

The study by Vecht *et al.* has been criticized for using a non-standard radiation dose (up to 40 Gray (Gy)/day). In addition in their study no magnetic resonance imaging (MRI) was used to confirm whether metastases were indeed solitary. Although 50% of patients with extracranial cancer will have a single brain metastasis detected on CT scan, this figure is reduced to 30% with MRI. It is possible, therefore, that in the study by Vecht *et al.* the patient population contained patients with >1 intracranial metastasis.

The study by Mintz *et al.* has been criticized by for including a large proportion of patients with active systemic disease and for differences in the distribution of histological diagnoses between the two groups (Wronski and Lederman, 1997). The surgical group containing tumours with poorer prognoses on the basis of histology (more colorectal primaries) compared to the radiation group (more breast tumours). However, the authors have refuted this as a potential source of bias arguing that the most important factor influencing survival was the extent of extracranial disease, not individual histology (Levine, 1997).

All three studies have been criticized for containing a variety of pathologies with different radiosensitivites. Ideally, a trial would include only radiosensitive tumours. Nevertheless, the trials reflect realistic clinical practice.

Further controlled studies are required to evaluate the role of surgery in different tumour types. In addition, there is a need for controlled studies evaluating the role of surgery in multiple cerebral metastases. However, these three trials have established the role of surgical resection as a treatment option in the management of patients with a single brain metastasis. It is significant that the trial by Mintz *et al.* appears to contradict the findings of the previous two trials. As has been mentioned above, the results of this third trial may have been influenced by the inclusion of patients with factors associated with a poor outcome with surgery. This led to a number of studies to assess the prognostic factors in patients with cerebral metastasis in order to facilitate the selection of good surgical candidates. The most important of these studies was carried out by the Radiation Therapy Oncology Group (RTOG), which developed the recursive partitioning analysis (RPA) classification on the basis of a retrospective study of 1200 patients. The RPA classification is a statistical method of classifying patients on the basis of several factors: KPS score; age; and extent of extracranial disease (Gaspar *et al.*, 1997). The RPA classification is as follows:

Class I	KPS ≥70
	age <65 years
	controlled primary tumour
	brain is only site of metastasis
Class II	KPS ≥70
	age >65 years
	uncontrolled systemic disease/other symptomatic metastases
Class III	KPS <70

In their study of 1200 patients treated with radiotherapy, the authors found that the median survival for the different classes was as follows: Class I (7.1 months); Class II (4.2 months); and Class III (2.3 months). The RPA classification has also been shown to have prognostic value in patients treated surgically (Agboola *et al.*, 1998). Class I patients are the group most likely to benefit from craniotomy, although it is important to consider the histology of the primary tumour as well, e.g. patients with metastasis from renal cell carcinoma or melanoma may have poorer survival rates than breast cancer metastasis (Sills, 2005). If RPA classification had been used in the three trials reviewed in this section it is possible that all three may have shown a beneficial effect of surgery. It is likely that RPA classification will be used in the design and analysis of future trials.

Agboola O, Benott B, Cross P, Da Silva V, Esche B, Lesuik H, Gonsalves C. Prognositc factors derived from recursive partition analysis (RPA) of radiation therapy oncology group (RTOG) brain metastasis trials applied to surgically resected and irradiated brain metastatic cases. *Int J Radiation Oncology Biol Phys* 1998; **42**: 155–159.

Cairncross JG, Jim JH, Posner JB. Radiation therapy for brain metastases. *Ann Neurol* 1980; **7**: 175–224.

Gaspar L, Scott C, Rotman M, Asbell S, Phillips T, Wasserman T, McKenna WG, Byhardt. Recursive partitioning analysis (RPA) of prognostic factors in three radiation therapy oncology group (RTOG) brain metastases trials. *In J Radiat Oncol Biol Phys* 1997; **37**: 745–751.

Levine M. Correspondence: a randomised trial to assess the efficacy of surgery in addition to radiotherapy in patients with a single cerebral metastasis – author reply. *Cancer* 1997; **80**: 1003–1004.

Posner JB. Surgery for metastases to the brain. *New Engl J Med* 1990; **322**: 544–545

Sills AK. Current treatment approaches to surgery for brain metastases. *Neurosurgery* 2005; **57**: S4–S24.

Wronski M, Lederman G. Correspondence: a randomised trial to assess the efficacy of surgery in addition to radiotherapy in patients with a single cerebral metastasis. *Cancer* 1997; **80**: 1002–1003.

2.3 **Adjuvant radiotherapy for single brain metastases**

Details of study

This study is the only RCT looking at WBRT as an adjunct to surgery. The study was carried out in Kentucky, United States in the 1990s.

Study references

Main study

Patchell RA, Tibbs PA, Regine WF, Dempsey RJ, Mohiuddin M, Kryscio RJ, Markesbery WR, Foon KA, Young B. Postoperative radiotherapy in the treatment of single metastases to the brain: a randomized trial. *JAMA* 1998; **280**: 1485–1489.

Related reference

Patchell RA, Regine WF. The rationale for adjuvant whole brain radiation therapy with radiosurgery in the treatment of single brain metastases. *Technol Cancer Res Treat* 2003; **2**: 111–115.

Study design

* Multi-centre, parallel group RCT

Class of evidence	I
Randomization	Surgery versus surgery + WBRT
Number of patients	95
Follow-up	Life span of patients
	Primary endpoint: Recurrence of tumour
	Secondary endpoints: Survival Cause of death Functional independence
Number of centres	>1 (unspecified)
Stratification	Extent of disease Primary tumour type

* Inclusion criteria: Patients >18 with single metastasis completely resected.

* Exclusion criteria: Incomplete resection; leptomeningeal metastases; previous radiotherapy; other malignancy; KPS <70; need for emergency surgery; highly radiosensitive primary tumours (e.g. small cell lung cancer).

* MRIs were carried out to establish the presence of single metastases.

* DXT started within 28 days of surgery.

* Intention-to-treat analysis.

Outcome measures

Primary endpoints

- Recurrence of metastases: 3-monthly MRIs for the first year and then 6-monthly; recurrence divided into original (site of resection) or distant (other site in brain).

Secondary endpoints

- Length of survival
- Cause of death
- Functional independence: defined as period of time with KPS >70

Results

		Surgery alone	Surgery + WBRT	Statistical significance
Original recurrence	Rate	46%	10%	$p < 0.001$
	Time to recurrence	27 weeks	52 weeks	$p < 0.001$
Overall recurrence		70%	18%	$p < 0.001$
Median survival		43 weeks	46 weeks	None
Cause of death	Neurological	44%	14%	$p = 0.03$
	Systemic	46%	84%	$p < 0.001$
Length of functional independence		35 weeks	37 weeks	None

Conclusions

Routine post-operative WBRT reduces recurrence of brain metastases and reduces death from neurological causes.

Critique

This trial is unique as WBRT is an established treatment for brain metastases. Indeed, the trial has been criticized for looking at a somewhat unconventional approach for the management of brain metastases. However, the use of WBRT as an adjuvant therapy had been looked at in clinical series but no clinical trial had previously been carried out. Following their study reported in 1990 looking at surgery plus WBRT versus WBRT alone, the question as to whether WBRT after surgery has any benefit remained to be addressed by way of a RCT.

The primary endpoint of this trial was recurrence of metastasis in the brain and the trial size was based on answering this question. The trial was not powered to make conclusions regarding survival. The results need to be interpreted, therefore, with this in mind. Certainly, the results showed that the recurrence of the brain metastasis was significantly lower in those receiving post-operative WBRT. There was no difference in overall mortality in patients receiving surgery alone versus those receiving post-operative DXT. However, patients in the surgery plus DXT group were much more likely to die from systemic causes, while those in the DXT group were much likely to die from neurological causes. Although the trial was not large enough to extrapolate these findings to the wider population, the findings are in keeping with the previous trial by Patchell *et al.*, which looked at WBRT with or without surgery in these patients (Patchell *et al.*, 1990). It appears, therefore, that treatment focused on the single brain metastasis may well reduce the incidence of death from brain disease. This finding suggests that the treatment arms alter the mode of but not the time of death and begs the question as to whether one cause of death is more acceptable by another to patients and their families.

Patchell *et al.* concluded that their results supported the routine use of WBRT in patients with single brain metastases. However, it has been pointed out that a subset of patients in the surgery group who died of systemic causes had the longest median survival of 88 weeks and this would suggest that DXT may be detrimental in this subgroup of patients (Carol and Rosa, 1999). Nonetheless, this criticism is based on a post-hoc analysis of a small number of patients only and Patchell *et al.* have emphasized that the primary endpoint of their study was recurrence of the original brain metastasis and not survival (Patchell *et al.*, 1999).

This study by Patchell *et al.* is the only randomized prospective study evaluating the role of WBRT as an adjuvant treatment to surgical resection and as such is a landmark study in neuro-oncology.

Carol W, Rosa S. Letters to the editor. *JAMA* 1999; **281**: 1695.

Patchell RA, Tibbs PA, Regine WF, Mohiuddin M, Kryscia RH, Markesbery WR, Foon KA, Young B, Dempsey RJ. Author reply. *JAMA* 1999; **281**: 1696.

2.4 **Stereotactic radiosurgery for brain metastases**

Details of studies

Two multi-centre randomized trials have been carried out to evaluate the role of stereotactic radiosurgery in the management of cerebral metastases. The first trial, carried out by RTOG in North America between 1996 and 2001, compared WBRT with or without stereotactic radiosurgery (SRS) in patients with one to three metastases. The second trial, carried out by the Japanese Radiation Oncology Study Group (JROSG) in Japan between 1999 and 2004, compared SRS with or without WBRT in patients with one to four metastases.

Study references

Main studies

Andrews DW, Scott CB, Sperduto PW, Flanders AE, Gaspar LE, Schell MC, Werner-Wasik M, Demas W, Ryu J, Bahary JP, Souhami L, Rotman M, Mehta MP, Curran WJ Jr. Whole brain radiation therapy with or without stereotactic radiosurgery boost for patients with one to three brain metastases: phase III results of the RTOG 9508 randomised trial. *Lancet* 2004; **363**: 1655–1672.

Aoyama H, Shirato H, Tago T, Nakagawa K, Toyoda T, Hatano K, Kenjyo M, Oya N, Hirota S, Shioura H, Kunieda E, Inomata T, Hayakawa K, Katoh N, Kobashi G. Stereotactic radiosurgery plus whole-brain radiatin therapy vs stereotactic radiosurgery alone for the treatment of brain metastases – a randomised controlled trial. *JAMA* 2006; **21**: 2483–2491.

Related reference

Raizer J. Radiosurgery and whole-brain radiation therapy for brain metastases either both or as the optimal treatment. *JAMA* 2006; **295**: 2535–2536.

Study design

	RTOG trial	JRSOG trial
Class of evidence	I	I
Randomization	WBRT versus WBRT + SRS	SRS versus SRS +WBRT
Number of patients	333	132
Follow-up	100%	100%
	Primary endpoint: ◆ Survival	Primary endpoint: ◆ Overall survival
	Secondary endpoint: ◆ Tumour response ◆ Brain tumour recurrence ◆ Functional performance ◆ Cause of death	Secondary endpoints: ◆ Brain tumour recurrence ◆ Salvage brain treatment ◆ Functional preservation ◆ Toxic effects of radiation ◆ Cause of death
Number of centres	55	11
Stratification	◆ Number of brain metastases ◆ Extent of extracranial disease	◆ Number of brain metastases ◆ Extent of extracranial disease ◆ Primary tumour site (lung versus other sites)

- Intention-to-treat analyses used in both trials.
- RTOG eligibility
  - Inclusion criteria: Age ≥18 years; one to three brain metastases confirmed with contrast MRI; metastasis diameter ≤4 cm; KPS ≥70; consent.
  - Exclusion criteria: Brainstem metastases; active systemic disease; deranged haematology (e.g. low Hb, platelets or neutrophil count); RPA class III.
- JRSOG eligibility
  - Inclusion criteria: Age ≥18 years; one to four brain metastases confirmed with contrast MRI; metastasis diameter ≤3 cm; histological confirmation of systemic disease; KPS ≥70; consent.
  - Exclusion criteria: Small cell lung carcinoma; lymphoma; germinoma; multiple myeloma.
- Patients in the RTOG study all received WBRT in daily 2.5 Gy fractions to a total of 37.5 Gy with SRS doses varying according to the size of the metastases.
- Patients in the JRSOG study who received WBRT were given 10 fractions to a total of 30 Gy and SRS doses varied according to size of the metastases.

Results

Overall survival

	RTOG trial			JRSOG trial			
	WBRT	WBRT + SRS	Statistical significance		SRS	SRS + WBRT	Statistical significance
Mean Survival time	6.5 months	5.7 months	None	Median survival	8 months	7.5 months	None

- In the RTOG trial, a survival benefit was found with the addition of SRS to WBRT in those patients with a single brain metastasis: mean survival time in the WBRT + SRS group was 6.5 months compared to 4.9 months in the WBRT-alone group ($p < 0.04$).

Brain tumour recurrence

- RTOG trial: Radiological evaluation at 1 year revealed better control in the WBRT plus SRS group (82%) than in the WBRT-alone group (71%, $p = 0.01$). However, this evaluation was carried out in <23% of the enrolled patients.
- JRSOG trial: Recurrence rate at 12 months was much greater in the SRS-alone group (76.4%) than in the SRS plus WBRT group (46.8%; $p < 0.001$).

Functional performance

- RTOG trial: KPS scores were more likely to have improved at 6 months follow-up in the WBRT plus SRS group (43%) than in the WBRT-alone group (27%, $p = 0.03$).

- JRSOG trial: Although no significant differences in KPS scores were found between groups it is noteworthy that significantly more patients in the SRS-alone group (86%) showed neurological deterioration attributable to progression of brain metastases than those in the SRS plus WBRT group (59%, $p= 0.05$).

Cause of death

- No significant differences in the causes of death (neurological versus non-neurological) were found between the groups in either study.

Conclusions

RTOG trial

- An SRS boost following WBRT is better than WBRT alone for single brain metastasis and should be a standard treatment for all patients with a single brain metastasis.
- An SRS boost following WBRT improves performance in all patients with up to three brain metastases and should be considered for all patients with two to three brain metastases.

JRSOG trial

- The addition of WBRT to SRS does not improve survival in patients with brain metastases.
- Intracranial relapse was more likely with SRS alone, but without increased risk of neurologic death.

Critique

Intracranial metastases occur in approximately one-third of patients with cancer. WBRT has been the mainstay of treatment for brain metastases with surgery. The rationale for WBRT is based on the assumption that haematogenous spread of the primary tumour has seeded the whole brain and that, in addition to macroscopic metastases, there will be microscopic metastases that will remain occult on conventional neuroimaging modalities such as computed tomography (CT) and MRI. However, an alternative view is that intracranial disease may be actually locally limited. Certainly, surgery appears to be beneficial in patients with single metastases who are good surgical candidates. However, the majority of patients will have multiple metastases and SRS has several potential advantages that may be beneficial in this situation. SRS allows for the focal administration of high-dose radiation to multiple lesions including some that may be otherwise surgically inaccessible. In addition, SRS may potentially reduce the neurotoxic effects of WBRT if it is effective. The two trials considered here have taken different approaches to evaluate the effects of SRS in the management of cerebral metastases. The RTOG study evaluated the addition of SRS to conventional WBRT, whereas the JRSOG study took the alternative approach of evaluating the addition of WBRT to SRS therapy. In this way, the JRSOG study has some philosophical similarities with the study by Patchell *et al.*, which considered the addition of WBRT to surgery for single brain metastasis (Patchell *et al.*, 1998). However, Patchell and colleagues have published one of the more unforgiving critical appraisals of the JRSOG study in which they raise several points of contention (Patchell *et al.*, 2006). They argue that as it was unlikely that any survival difference would be seen between the two groups, it was incorrect to conduct power calculations on the basis of a potential survival benefit. They propose that the study should have been powered to calculate non-inferiority of SRS alone and that this would have required the recruitment of 17-fold more patients than are actually included in the study, indicating that the JRSOG study is grossly underpowered. The view of Patchell *et al.* is that the only statistically supported finding in the JRSOG trial is that the addition of WBRT to SRS reduces recurrence of brain metastases. They express the view, therefore, that the JRSOG supports the upfront use of WBRT, a conclusion that would be supported by the finding that less patients in the SRS plus WBRT suffered neurologic deterioration from tumour progression.

The RTOG trial may have been hindered by several factors, not the least of which was the inclusion of patients who had undergone surgical resection or brain metastases without any stratification. In addition, there was limited complete radiological follow-up of patients (less than half the patient population). Notwithstanding the limitations of these studies they are both landmark studies. The RTOG study is the first completed large multi-centre randomized trial evaluating the role of a SRS boost following WBRT for brain metastases. The JRSOG study, although subject to much criticism, has also added significantly to the debate regarding the role of SRS in the management of brain metastases. A phase III trial evaluating microsurgery plus WBRT versus SRS alone for single brain metastases was recently published but unfortunately due to patient accrual the study was discontinued early and so no conclusions could be drawn (Muacevic *et al.*, 2008). The role of SRS will be further elucidated with large well-designed multi-centre randomized trials.

Muacevic A, Wowra B, Siefert A, Tonn JG, Steiger HJ, Kreth FW. Microsurgery plus whole brain irradiation versus gamma knife surgery for treatment of single metastases to the brain: a randomised controlled multicentre phase III trial. *J Neurooncol* 2008; **87**: 299–307.

Patchell RA, Regine WF, Renschler M, Loeffler JS, Sawaya R, Chin LS, Andrews DW. Editorial: comments about the prospective randomised trial by Aoyama *et al*. *Surg Neurol* 2006; **66**: 459–460.

2.5 **Extent of resection of malignant glioma**

Details of studies

Numerous clinical series have evaluated the relationship between the extent of resection and survival in patients with malignant glioma. Although 'total' resection appears to prolong life more than subtotal resection, it may be that this reflects a selection bias towards younger, fitter patients with tumours in non-eloquent regions for more aggressive surgery. The advent of CT and MRI has allowed for the more accurate assessment of the extent of tumour resection. Three studies have been selected for inclusion here. The first is one of the earlier, larger, and better retrospective analyses of patients undergoing surgery for malignant glioma and was carried out at the Washington Medical Center in Seattle (Keles *et al.*, 1999). The second is the only RCT that compares biopsy with resection and was carried out in Finland (Vuorinen *et al.*, 2003). The third is the first multicentre RCT comparing two different methods of surgical resection (fluorescence-assisted surgery and conventional surgery) for malignant glioma and was carried out in Germany (Stummer *et al.*, 2006).

Study reference

Main studies

Keles GE, Anderson B, Berger MS. The effect of extent of resection on time to tumor progression and survival in patients with glioblastoma mulitforme of the cerebral hemisphere. *Cancer* 1999; **74**: 1784–1791.

Vuorinen V, Hinkka S, Farkilla M, Jasskelainen J. Debulking or biopsy of malignant glioma in elderly people – a randomized study. *Acta Neurochir (Wein)* 2003; **145**: 5–10.

Stummer W, Pichlmeier U, Meinel T, Wiestler OD, Zanella F, Reulen HJ; ALA-Glioma Study Group. Flourescence-guided surgery with 5-alaminovulinic acid for resection of malignant glioma: a randomised controlled mulitcentre phase III trial. *Lancet Oncol* 2006; **7**: 392–401

Related reference

Stummer W, Reulen HJ, Meinel T, Pichlmeier U, Schumacher W, Tonn JC, Rohde V, Oppel F, Turowski B, Woiciechowsky C, Franz K, Pietsch T; ALA-Glioma Study Group. Extent of resection and survival in glioblastoma multiforme: identification of and adjustment for bias. *Lancet Oncol* 2008; **7**: 392–401.

Study designs

1 Keles *et al.* (1999): Retrospective series analysis

2 Vuorinen *et al.* (2003): RCT

3 Stummer *et al.* (2006): RCT

	Keles *et al.* (1999)	Vuorinen *et al.* (2003)	Stummer *et al.* (2006)
Class of evidence	II	I	I
Randomization	None	Biopsy versus resection	Fluorescence-assisted surgery versus conventional surgery
Number of patients	92	30	322 (270 in analysis)

	Keles *et al.* (1999)	Vuorinen *et al.* (2003)	Stummer *et al.* (2006)
Follow-up	Life span of patients	Life span of patients	6 months
	Primary endpoints: Time to progression (TTP) Survival	Primary endpoints: Survival	Primary endpoints: Progression-free survival (PFS) Degree of resection
	Other endpoints: None	Other endpoints: Clinical status KPS	Other endpoints: Volume of residual tumour Overall survival Neurological deficit Toxicity
Number of centres	1	1	17
Stratification	None	None	None

Keles *et al.* (1999)

- Radiological extent of resection was assessed by examining and making volumetric measurements of pre-operative and post-operative CTs and/or MRI.
- Strict inclusion criteria were used to reduce variables that might bias the prognosis: Adult patients with KPS >70 and glioblastoma multiforme in a cerebral hemisphere.

Vuorinen *et al.* (2003)

- Inclusion criteria: Radiological diagnosis of malignant glioma (supratentorial); KPS >60; age >65; informed consent.
- All patients received radiotherapy unless their clinical state deteriorated too far.
- Intention-to-treat analysis.

Stummer *et al.* (2006)

- Total resection was defined as no contrast-enhancing tumour on MRI at 72 h post-operatively.
- Fluorescence was achieved by the pre-operative administration of 5-aminolevulinic acid (5-ALA).
- Conventional surgery was performed under white light.
- PFS at 6 months was assessed with MRI.
- The study was terminated early and 270 patients were included in the analysis.

Results

Keles *et al.* (1999)

Extent of resection	<25%	25–49%	50–74%	75–99%	100%
Median TTP (weeks)	14.1	24	31.9	45.8	53.1
Median survival (weeks)	31.8	56.6	62.9	88.5	93

- Extent of resection also showed a significant correlation with post-operative KPS ($p < 0.05$).

Vuorinen *et al.* (2003)

	Craniotomy and resection	Biopsy	Statistical significance
Median survival (days)	171	85	$p = 0.03$
PFS (6 months)	41%	21%	$p = 0.0003$

- There was a survival advantage of >2 months for craniotomy and surgical resection ($p < 0.05$).

Stummer *et al.* (2006)

	Fluorescence-assisted surgery	Conventional surgery	Statistical significance
Percentage of complete resections	65%	36%	$p < 0.0001$
PFS (6 months)	41%	21%	$p = 0.0003$

Conclusions

Keles *et al.* (1999)

The extent of tumour resection of glioblastoma multiforme affects overall survival and time to progression.

Vuorinen *et al.* (2003)

Craniotomy and debulking offers a modest survival advantage over biopsy in elderly patients with malignant gliomas.

Stummer *et al.* (2006)

Fluorescence-assisted surgery with 5-ALA enables more complete resection of malignant gliomas with improved progression-free survival.

Critique

Although the study by Keles and colleagues is only a retrospective series it is to be commended because it attempts to reduce the effect of selection bias by using strict inclusion criteria. In addition, the authors have used radiological assessments of the extent of tumour resection rather than estimates by the operating surgeon. The study was restricted to glioblastoma multiforme and not all high-grade gliomas. Nonetheless, the results of this study are informative and may be generally representative of the effects of the extent of resection in high-grade gliomas. Indeed, a larger, more recent multivariate analysis has also found that gross-total tumour resection is associated with longer survival (Lacroix et al., 2001). The study by Keles and colleagues still stands out as a landmark in the retrospective series because of their use of radiological measures of tumour resection and efforts to reduce bias from other prognostic variable.

The study by Vuorinen and colleagues is hindered by the small numbers of patients and the fact that they are elderly. However, the reason why the patients were >65 years of age was that the authors felt there was most equipoise in this group regarding biopsy or resection. It would not be prudent, therefore, to suggest that the results of this small trial would necessarily reflect the situation in the more general population. Nonetheless, the results are in keeping with the widespread and long-standing presumption that extent of resection is likely to be a prognostic factor in malignant glioma patients, and the study is a landmark as it randomized to try to answer this fundamental question.

By comparing the two methods of tumour resection, Stummer and colleagues have been able to perform the first RCT in this area. Although the nature of the two surgical techniques does not allow a blind study to be performed, the trial still stands out as the first trial of its kind. In a subsequent analysis, the authors have been able to compare survival rates in patients with and without 'complete' resection ('complete' according to their radiological definition). They report that survival is greater in patients with 'complete' resection (16.7 versus 11.8 months, $p < 0.0001$). The authors assert that their trial is Level II evidence that 'complete' resection is associated with improved survival in malignant glioma. However, it should be noted that the trial is a comparison of two techniques rather than randomization of extent of resection.

Lacroix M, Abi-Said D, Fourney DR, Gokaslan ZL, Shi W, DeMonte F, Lang FF, McCutcheon IE, Hassenbusch SJ, Holland E, Hess K, Michael C, Miller D, Sawaya R. A multivariate analysis of 416 patients with glioblastoma multiforme: prognosis, extent of resection, and survival. *J Neurosurg* 2001; 95: 190–198.

Stummer W, Reulen HJ, Meinel T, Pichlmeier U, Schumacher W, Tonn JC, Rohde V, Oppel F, Turowski B, Woiciechowsky C, Franz K, Pietsch T; ALA-Glioma Study Group. Extent of resection and survival in glioblastoma multiforme: identification of and adjustment for bias. *Lancet Oncol* 2006; 7: 392–401.

2.6 **Early concomitant systemic chemotherapy with radiotherapy for glioblastoma**

Details of study

The role of systemic temozolomide chemotherapy for glioblastoma was evaluated by the EORTC and the NCIC and is familiarly known as the 'temozolomide trial' (Stupp *et al.*, 2005). This trial was carried out in Europe and North America between 2000 and 2002 and has led to the routine use of temozolomide chemotherapy in patients with glioblastomas.

Study references

Main study

Stupp R, Mason WP, van den Bent MJ, Weller M, Fisher B, Taphoorn MJB, Belander K, Brande AA, Marosi C, Bogdahn U, Curschmann K, janzer RC, Ludwin SK, Gorlia T, Allgeier A, Lacombe D, Cairncross G, Eisenhauer E, Mirimanoff RO, for the European Organisation for Research and Treatment of Cancer Brain Tumour and Radiotherapy Groups and the National Institute of Canada Clinical Trials Group. Radiotherapy plus concomitant and adjuvant temozolomide for glioblastoma. *N Engl J Med* 2005; **352**: 987–996.

Related reference

Hegi R, Diserens AC, Gorlia T, Hamou MF, de Tribolet N, Weller M, Kros JM, Hainfellner JA, Mason W, Mariani L, Bromberg JEC, Hau P, Mirimanoff RO, Cairncross G, Janzer RC, Stupp R. MGMT gene silencing and benefit from temozolomide in glioblastoma. *N Engl J Med* 2005; **352**: 997–1003.

Study design

* A prospective multi-institutional RCT

Class of evidence	I
Randomization	DXT alone versus DXT + temozolomide
Number of patients	573
Follow-up	Life span of patients
	Primary endpoint: Overall survival
	Secondary endpoints: Quality of life Safety Progression-free survival
Number of centres	85 centres in 15 countries
Stratification	WHO performance status

* Inclusion criteria: Newly diagnosed glioblastoma multiforme (GBM); age 18–70; 'good clinical state'; consent.

- A total of 60 Gy radiotherapy was administered in daily 2 Gy fractions over 6 weeks (5 days per week).
- Patients in the temozolomide arm were also given continuous daily temozolomide (75 mg/m^2 of body surface area per day) for the duration of the radiotherapy and this was followed by six adjuvant cycles of temozolomide (150–200 mg/m^2 for 5 days during every 28-day cycle).

Outcome measures

Primary endpoint
- Overall survival was analysed using the Kaplan–Meier method.

Secondary endpoints
- Safety: Patients were evaluated regularly for adverse events including haematological monitoring.
- Quality of life questionnaires were also used during regular follow-up.
- Progression-free survival was also analysed using the Kaplan–Meier method.

Results
- The median age of patients was 56 years and 86% underwent debulking surgery.
- Ninety-three percent of patients had a histological confirmation of glioblastoma.

	DXT + temozolomide	DXT alone	Statistical significance
Median survival	14.6 months	12.1 months	$p < 0.001$
Median progression-free survival	6.9 months	5 months	$p < 0.001$

- The relative reduction in risk of death in patients receiving temozolomide was 37% (hazard ratio of 0.63 compared to the DXT-alone group).
- The hazard ratio for death or disease progression in the temozolomide group compared to the DXT-alone group was 0.54.
- Two-year survival rates were greater in the temozolomide group (26.5%) compared to the DXT-alone group (10.4%).
- A translational study found that O^6-methylguanine-DNA methyltransferase (MGMT) promotor methylation is associated with a survival benefit for temozolomide + DXT (21 months versus 15 months, $p < 0.05$).
- There were no significant differences in the safety profiles of each treatment arm.
- There was no adverse effect on quality of life by the addition of temozolomide therapy.
- Subgroup analysis did not reveal any difference in survival advantage between subgroups.

Conclusions

The early addition of temozolomide chemotherapy to radiotherapy has a significant survival advantage in patients with glioblastoma.

Critique

Chemotherapy given before, or as an adjuvant to radiotherapy has been evaluated in multiple clinical trials and found to have minimal impact on survival in patients with glioblastoma (Fine *et al.*, 1993; Stewart, 2002). This temozolomide trial addressed the question as to whether early addition of temozolomide chemotherapy to radiotherapy would have any advantage over radiotherapy alone. The concomitant use of a chemotherapeutic agent with radiotherapy was an unconventional approach and this is a landmark study as it reports the greatest improvement in survival (more than 50%) in patients with glioblastoma since the trial of radiotherapy versus chemotherapy with an alkylating agent over a quarter of a century earlier (Walker *et al.*, 1978). This may reflect the selection of patients with good prognostic indicators (tumour resection, young age, good functional status) and the less toxic effects of temozolomide compared to other nitrosourea-based chemotherapeutic agents. The beneficial effects of temozolomide have more recently been reported to last up to 5 years (Stupp *et al.*, 2009).

The translational study by Hegi *et al.* found that methylation of the MGMT promoter was associated with an even greater survival advantage. However, the clear survival advantage seen for all patients receiving temozolomide would appear to negate the value of reserving temozolomide for patients in this subgroup alone and so this study does not necessarily have the same impact as molecular genetic classification of oligodendrogliomas has had (Cairncross *et al.*, 1998).

The temozolomide trial demonstrates a survival benefit with low toxicity and has led to a new standard of care in patients with malignant glioma (Mason and Cairncross, 2005).

Cairncross JG, Ueki K, Zlatescu MC, Lisle DK, Finkelstein DM, Hammond RR, Silver JS, Stark PC, Macdonald DR, Ino Y, Ramsay DA, Louis DN. Specific genetic predictors of chemotherapeutic response and survival in patients with anaplastic oligodendrogliomas. *J Natl Cancer Inst* 1998; **90**: 1473–1479.

Fine HA, Dear KB, Loeffer JS, Black PM, Canellos GP. Meta-analysis of radiation therapy with and without adjuvant chemotherapy for malignant gliomas in adults. *Cancer* 1993; **71**: 2585–2597.

Mason WP, Cairncross JG. Drug Insight: temozolomide as a treatment for malignant glioma – impact of a recent trial. *Nat Clin Pract Neurol* 2005; **1**: 88–95.

Stewart LA. Chemotherapy in adult high-grade glioma: a systematic review and meta-analysis of individual patient data from 12 randomised trials. *Lancet* 2002; **359**: 1011–1018.

Stupp R, Hegi ME, Mason WP, van den Bent MJ, Taphoorn MJ, Janzer RC, Ludwin SK, Allgeier A, Fisher B, Belanger K, Hau P, Brandes AA, Gijtenbeek J, Marosi C, Vecht CJ, Mokhtari K, Wesseling P, Villa S, Eisenhauer E, Gorila T, Weller M, Lacombe D, Cairncross JG, Mirimanoff RO; European Organisation for Research and Treatment of Cancer Brain Tumour and Radiation Oncology Groups; National Cancer Institute of Canada Clinical trails Group. Effects of radiotherapy with concomitant and adjuvant temozolomide versus radiotherapy alone on survival in glioblastoma in a randomised phase III study: 5-year analysis of the EORTC-NCIC trail. *Lancet Oncol* 2009; **10**: 459–466.

Walker MD, Alexanderander E Jr, Hunt WE, MacCarty CS, Mahaley MS Jr, Mealey J Jr, Norrell HA, Owens G, Ransohoff J, Wilson CB, Gehan EA, Strike TA. Evaluation of BCNU and/or radiotherapy in the treatment of anaplastic gliomas. A cooperative clinical trial. *J Neurosurg* 1978; **49**: 333–343.

2.7 **Adjuvant localized chemotherapy (carmustine wafers) for malignant gliomas**

Details of studies

Three randomized controlled trials have been carried out to evaluate the effect of local administration of carmustine wafers to the tumour site in patients with malignant gliomas. The first was performed in the United States between 1989 and 1993 by the Polymer-Brain Tumor Treatment Group (PBTTG) and evaluated their efficacy against placebo in the treatment of recurrent glioblastomas requiring reoperation (Brem *et al.*, 1995). The second trial, which was carried out in Finland between 1992 and 1993, was designed to evaluate the efficacy of carmustine wafers applied at the time of the first operation (Valtonen *et al.*, 1997). Unfortunately, this trial included only a small number of patients and was discontinued early because of difficulties in availability of carmustine wafers. However, a third much larger trial, carried out by the Gliadel Study Group (GSG) in both North America and Europe between 1997 and 2000, also evaluated the efficacy of carmustine wafers applied to the resection cavity (Westphal *et al.*, 2003). A further long-term follow-up of this trial has also been published (Westphal *et al.*, 2006). The PBTTG and GSG trials are summarized here.

Study references

Main studies

Brem H, Piantadosi S, Burger PC, Walker M, Selker R, Vick NA, Black K, Sisti M, Brem S, Mohr G, Muller P, Morawetz R, Schold SC, for the Polymer-Brain Tumor Treatment Group. Placebo-controlled trial of safety and efficacy of intraoperative controlled delivery by biodegradable polymers of chemotherapy for recurrent gliomas. *Lancet* 1995; **345**: 1008–1012.

Westphal M, Hilt DC, Bortey E, Delavault P, Olivaras R, Warnke PC, Whittle IR, Jääskeläinen J, Ram Z. A phase 3 trial of local chemotherapy with biodegradable carmustine (BCNU) wafers (Gliadel wafers) in patients with primary malignant glioma. *Neuro-Oncology* 2003; **5**: 79–88.

Westphal M, Ram Z, Riddle V, Hilt D, Bortey E. Gliadel wafer in initial surgery for malignant glioma: long-term follow-up of a multi-center controlled trial. *Acta Neurochir (Wein)* 2006; **148**: 269–275.

Related reference

Valtonen S, Timonen U, Toivanen P, Kalimo H, Kivipelto L, Heiskanen O, Unsgaard G, Kuume T. Interstitial chemotherapy with carmustine with carmustine-loaded polymers for high-grade gliomas: a randomised double-blind study. *Neurosurgery* 1997; **41**: 44–48.

Study designs

◆ Both multi-centre, double-blind PRCTs

	PBTTG trial (Recurrent high-grade gliomas)	**GSG trial** (Primary high-grade gliomas)
Class of evidence	I	I
Randomization	Carmustine versus placebo	Carmustine versus placebo
Number of patients	222	240

	PBTTG trial (Recurrent high-grade gliomas)	GSG trial (Primary high-grade gliomas)
Follow-up	30 months (extened to 56 months on long-term follow-up)	At least 6 months and lifetime of patients
	Primary endpoint: Survival	Primary endpoint: Overall survival at 12 months
	Secondary endpoints: Complications Toxicity Quality of life	Secondary endpoint: Disease progression Quality of life Safety
Number of centres	27	38 (in 14 countries)
Stratification	Institution	Study centre Country

PBTTG trial

◆ Inclusion criteria: Unilateral tumour (size ≥1 cm on contrast-CT); KPS ≥60; completion of DXT; no nitrosoureas in previous 6 weeks; independent surgical decision on need for recurrent surgery.

◆ A proportional hazards regression model was used for statistical analysis in order to control for chance imbalances and differences in strong prognostic factors between groups.

◆ Intention-to-treat analysis.

GSG trial

◆ Inclusion criteria: Age 18–65; intra-operative frozen section confirming diagnosis of malignant glioma; KPS ≥60; radiological evidence of a single unilateral supratentorial tumour.

◆ The sample size of the trial was calculated to detect an 18% difference in 1-year survival between Gliadel and placebo (α level 0.05, power 0.90).

◆ A multiple regression analysis using the Cox proportional hazards model was used to account for effects of prognostic factors on survival.

◆ A secondary analysis was carried out for the glioblastoma subgroup although the trial was not designed to detect differences between histological subgroups.

Outcomes

◆ Kaplan–Meier curves were employed in both studies for the primary endpoints of survival.

Results

	PBTTG trial			GSG trial		
	Carmustine wafer	Placebo	Statistical significance	Carmustine wafer	Placebo	Statistical significance
Overall survival	60% (at 6 months)	47% (at 6 months)	None	59.2% (at 1 year)	49.2% (at 1 year)	$p < 0.05$
Median survival	31 weeks	23 weeks	$p = 0.006*$	13.8 months	11.6 months	$p = 0.017$

* After adjusting for prognostic factors.

PBTTG trial

- No statistically significant effect of carmustine wafers was found in the primary analysis.
- A treatment effect was seen for carmustine wafers only once adjustment had been made for the effects of prognostic factors: >75% resection; KPS >70; young age.
- Subgroup analysis of patients with GBM showed an apparent 6-month survival advantage for patients with carmustine over placebo (carmustine group 56%, placebo 36%, $p = 0.02$).
- There was no significant difference in adverse events between the two groups.

GSG trial

- Survival benefits remained significant at 3-year follow-up (carmustine group 9.2%, placebo group 1.7%, $p = 0.01$).
- Hazard ratio was 0.73 ($p = 0.018$) representing a 27% risk reduction.
- A subgroup analysis of patients with GBM did not reveal a statistically significant median survival benefit for carmustine (carmustine group 13.1 months, placebo group 11.4 months, $p = 0.08$).
- There was no significant difference in adverse events between the two groups.

Conclusions

GSG trial: Newly diagnosed malignant glioma patients benefit from carmustine wafers applied to the resection cavity at first operation.

Critique

The rationale for local delivery of a chemotherapeutic agent to glioblastomas is to combat local recurrence, avoid systemic side effects and to circumvent the blood–brain barrier.

Primary analysis in the PBTG trial by Brem *et al.* did not reveal a benefit for the carmustine wafers over placebo in patients with recurrent malignant gliomas. However, a statistically significant survival advantage was apparent in a subgroup analysis of patients with GBM and in the overall patient population once strong prognostic indicators were taken into account. However, conclusions from these post-hoc analyses have been interpreted with caution as the study was not stratified for prognostic indicators or histological subgroups. Nevertheless, the work by Brem *et al.* stands out as a landmark by demonstrating the potential benefits of a new treatment strategy without significantly more adverse effects than conventional treatment regimes.

The GSG trial by Westphal *et al.* showed a 2-month survival advantage for patients with newly diagnosed malignant gliomas receiving carmustine wafers to the resection cavity at primary resection. No statistically significant survival benefit was seen in a subgroup analysis for patients with GBM. However, as with similar analyses in the trial by Brem *et al.* this was a post-hoc analysis and the trial had not been stratified for histological subgroups. The GSG trial has defined the potential benefits of carmustine wafers in patients with primary malignant glioma (Perry *et al.*, 2007). Further experience and future studies will help determine the patients most likely to benefit from this treatment and whether it is effective when combined with concomitant temozolomide and radiotherapy.

Perry J, Chambers A, Spithoff K, Laperriere N. Gliadel wafers in the treatment of malignant glioma: a systematic review. *Curr Oncol* 2007; **14**: 189–194.

2.8 Brachytherapy for malignant gliomas

Details of studies

There have been a number of series reporting the efficacy of brachytherapy or interstitial radiotherapy in the treatment of newly diagnosed and recurrent malignant gliomas. To date, however, there have been only two randomized trials. The first study was by the University of Toronto group (Laperriere *et al.*, 1998) while the second one was by the Brain Tumor Cooperative Group in the United States (Selker *et al.*, 2002).

Study references

Main studies

Laperriere NJ, Leung PM, McKenzie S, Milosevic M, Wong S, Glen J, Pintilie M, Bernstein M. Randomized study of brachytherapy in the initial management of patients with malignant astrocytoma. *Int J Radiat Oncol Biol Phys* 1998; **41**: 1005–1011.

Selker RG, Shapiro WR, Burger P, Blackwood MS, Deutsch M, Arena VA, Van Gilder JC, Wu J, Malkin MG, Mealey J, Neal JH, Olson J, Robertson JT, Barnett GH, Bloomfield S, Albright R, Hochberg FH, Hiesiger E, Green S. The Brain Tumor Cooperative Group NIH Trial 87-01: A randomized comparison of surgery, external radiotherapy, and carmustine versus surgery, interstitial radiotherapy boost, external radiation therapy, and carmustine. *Neurosurgery* 2002; **51**: 343–357.

Study designs

- All RCTs

Study	Laperriere *et al.* (1998)	Selker *et al.* (2002)
Class of evidence	I	I
Randomization	EBRT* versus EBRT + brachytherapy with I^{125} implants	Brachytherapy with I^{125} implants + EBRT + BCNU versus EBRT + BCNU
Number of patients	140	270
Follow-up	Life span of patient	3 years
	Primary endpoint: Overall survival from the date of initial surgery	Primary endpoint: Survival time from date of randomization
	Secondary endpoints: Quality of life KPS Steroid usage Tumour recurrence	Secondary endpoint: KPS Tumour recurrence
Number of centres	1	14
Stratification	Age KPS	Institution Age Extent of surgery KPS

*EBRT = external beam radiation therapy.

- Histopathological diagnosis was obtained through surgery, either biopsy or subtotal resection of the tumour.
- Both studies utilized stereotactically implanted high-activity I^{125} seeds to deliver brachytherapy. The total radiation dose delivered was 60 Gy to the tumour perimeter.
- Laperriere's group utilized conventional external beam radiation therapy (EBRT) on all enhancing tumour plus a 2.5-cm margin of surrounding brain. The prescribed dose was 50 Gy to the midplane in 25 fractions in 5 weeks.
- Selker's group utilized WBRT 43 Gy in 25 fractions plus a coned-down boost to the tumour volume for the first 64 patients. Subsequent patients received 60.2 Gy in 35 fractions to the tumour border plus a 3-cm margin.
- The chemotherapeutic agent used by Selker's group was 1, 3-bis (2-chloroethy 1)-1-nitrosourea (BCNU). It was administered intravenously at 200 mg/m^2 and given every 8 weeks until the course was completed or if the patient developed adverse effects.
- Extent of resection and tumour recurrence were determined by contrast-enhanced CT scan.

Inclusion and exclusion criteria

	Laperriere et al. (1998)	Selker et al. (2002)
Inclusion criteria	• Biopsy-proven supratentorial malignant astrocytoma of the brain • Maximum tumour diameter < or = 6 cm • No involvement of the corpus callosum • Age 18–70 • KPS > or = 70	• Age > 15 • Good KPS • Biopsy-proven supratentorial malignant glioma
Exclusion criteria	• Tumour diameter > 6 cm • Corpus callosum involved • Poor KPS	• Midline cross-over in the corpus callosum or other midline structures • Multicentric tumours • Absence of a contrast-enhancing 'target' after surgery • Age < 15 • Other known primary malignancies • KPS < 50 in the immediate 3-week postoperative period • Inability to effect a surgical resection, if indicated

Outcome measures

Primary outcomes

- Survival

Secondary outcomes

Laperriere *et al.* (1998)

- Quality of life determined by linear analogue self-report scales
- KPS
- Steroid usage
- Tumour recurrence

Selker *et al.* (2002)

- KPS
- Tumour recurrence

Results

Median survival

	Laperiere *et al.* (1998)			Selker *et al.* (2002)		
Treatment	EBRT	EBRT + I^{125}	Statistical significance	I^{125} + EBRT + BCNU	EBRT + BCNU	Statistical significance
Median survival	13.2 months	13.8 months	None ($p = 0.49$)	16 months	13.7 months	None ($p = 0.10$)

Other significant findings

Laperriere *et al.* (1998)

- There is a statistically significant increase in median dexamethasone dosage for patients on the implant arm of the study, although the KPS does not differ between the two arms of the study.
- Recurrence patterns vary between the two treatment groups. The non-implant arm shows a higher recurrence rate at the original site of the tumour, whereas the implant arm exhibits a higher incidence of multifocal recurrence.
- Prognostic factors that are associated with improved survival include age, performance status, chemotherapy at recurrence, and reoperation at recurrence.

Selker *et al.* (2002)

- Prognostic factors associated with improved survival include KPS, pathology (GBM versus non-GBM), sex, and age.

Conclusions

Both trials concluded that stereotactic radiation implants do not confer a survival advantage in patients with newly diagnosed malignant gliomas.

Critique

Brachytherapy is a form of radiotherapy delivered by implanting radioactive sources directly into the tumour. It delivers high doses of radiation to the tumour while sparing normal surrounding brain. Pathologic studies confirm that I^{125} brachytherapy decreases the proliferative capacity of the tumour (Siddiqi et al., 1997). However, this does not necessarily translate into clinical outcome such as improved survival.

Numerous series have been reported on the efficacy of brachytherapy (Davis, 1987; Kumar et al., 1989; Gutin et al., 1991; Hitchon et al., 1992; Prados et al., 1992), but these were all non-randomized studies with a high degree of patient selection. Brachytherapy has also been used for recurrent malignant gliomas (Bernstein et al., 1994) and recurrent brain metastases (Bernstein et al., 1995), but because of the small study populations, the results were inconclusive.

The main argument challenging the encouraging outcomes in the earlier brachytherapy studies is that the patients who were eligible for brachytherapy were younger and had a better performance status. In addition, their tumours were smaller, more peripherally located, and more circumscribed. The inherent characteristics of this subgroup may already be associated with a better prognosis despite the type of treatment given. The second argument is that patients who undergo brachytherapy may develop more significant radiation necrosis and thus, have a higher rate of reoperation to reduce the mass effect of the necrotic lesion and/or the tumour load. The additional survival may have been partly related to the beneficial effects of reoperation. Both arguments were put to rest by the RCTs discussed in this section. Both studies eliminated the effect of favourable patient and tumour characteristics by randomization, and both studies showed an equivalent number of reoperations in each group, which was not statistically significant.

Laperriere et al. can be criticized for using a dosage of 50 Gy during EBRT. At the time of the study, the optimal dose of EBRT for malignant gliomas had not been established, but the present recommendation is 60 Gy (Bleehen et al., 1991). However, this did not affect the design of the study because both treatment arms received the same dose of radiation.

Selker et al. implemented their study across 14 centres in the United States. This implies a wide variability in surgeon technical expertise and experience, and could affect the results of the study. The group also had a change in protocol with regard to EBRT: they utilized WBRT for the first 64 patients then modified their protocol afterwards to EBRT to the tumour plus a 3-cm margin. Although the group took into account this protocol change, with statistical analyses revealing that there is no difference in outcome between the patients who received the original versus the revised protocols, the actual effect in terms of amount of radiation necrosis and performance status may be unaccounted for.

Both studies utilized contrast-enhanced CT scans to plan dosimetry, measure the extent of resection, and detect tumour recurrence. During the active years of the study, MRI was still widely unavailable. It is not known whether using a better imaging modality such as MRI would affect the results of the study, but certainly it would give a more accurate estimate of the extent of resection and detect recurrent disease earlier.

Despite minor flaws, both studies are well designed and well executed. From the results, it is quite conclusive that brachytherapy has no role in the initial management of malignant glioma patients.

Bernstein M, Laperriere N, Glen J, Leung P, Thomason C, Landon AE. Brachytherapy for recurrent malignant astrocytoma. *Int J Radiat Oncol Biol Phys* 1994; **30**; 1213–1217.

Bernstein M, Cabantog A, Laperriere N, Leung P, Thomason C. Brachytherapy for recurrent single brain metastasis. *Can J Neurol Sci* 1995; **22**: 13–16.

Davis RL. Recurrent malignant gliomas: Survival following interstitial brachytherapy with high-activity iodine-125 sources. *J Neurosurg* 1987; **67**: 864–873.

Gutin PH, Prados MD, Phillips TL, Wara WM, Larson DA, Leibel SA, Sneed PK, Levine VA, Weaver KA, Silver P, Lamborn K, Lamb S, Ham RN. External irradiation followed by an interstitial high activity iodine-125 implant 'boost' in the initial treatment of malignant gliomas: NCOG Study 6G-82-2. *Int J Radiat Oncol Biol Phys* 1991; **21**; 601–606.

Hitchon PW, VanGilger JC, Wen BC, Jani S. Brachytherapy for malignant recurrent and untreated gliomas. *Stereo Funct Neurosurg* 1992; **59**: 174–178.

Kumar PP, Good RR, Jones EO, Patil AA, Leibrock LG, McComb RD. Survival of patients with glioblastoma multiforme treated by intraoperative high-activity cobalt 60 endocurietherapy. *Cancer* 1989; **64**: 1409–1413.

Prados MD, Gutin PH, Phillips TL, Wara WM, Sneed PK, Larson DA, Lamb SA, Ham B, Malec MK, Wilson CB. Interstitial brachytherapy for newly diagnosed patients with malignant gliomas: The UCSF experience. *Int J Radiat Oncol Biol Phys* 1992; **24**: 593–597.

Siddiqi SN, Provias J, Laperriere N, Bernstein M. Effects of iodine-125 brachytherapy on the proliferative capacity and histopathological features of glioblastoma recurring after initial therapy. *Neurosurgery* 1997; **40**: 910–917.

2.9 **Extent of resection of low-grade gliomas**
Details of studies

Two retrospective studies are included here which address the question of whether the extent of resection (EOR) of low-grade gliomas (LGG) affects outcome. The first study was carried out in San Francisco with the analysis of patients who underwent resection of LGG at the University of Calafornia, San Francisco between 1989 and 2005 (Smith *et al.*, 2008). The second was carried out in Baltimore with the analysis of patients who underwent resection LGG at the Johns Hopkins Department of Neurosurgery between 1996 and 2007 (McGirt *et al.*, 2008).

Study references
Main studies

McGirt MJ, Chaichana KL, Attenello FJ, Weingart JD, Than K, Burger P, Olivi AO, Brem H, Quinones-Hinojosa A. Extent of surgical resection is independently associated with survival in patients with hemispheric low-grade glioma. *Neurosurgery* 2008; **63**: 700–708.

Smith JS, Chang EF, Lamborn KR, Chang SM, Prados MD, Cha S, Tihan T, Vandenberg S. Role of extent of resection in the long-term outcome of low-grade hemispheric gliomas. *J Clin Oncol* 2008; **10**: 1338–1345.

Related reference

Laws ER Jr, Taylor WF, Clifton MB, Okazaki H. Neurosurgical management of low-grade astrocytoma of the cerebral hemispheres. *J Neurosurg* 1984; **61**: 665–673.

Study designs

♦ Both retrospective cohort studies

	Baltimore Group (McGirt *et al.*)	San Francisco Group (Smith *et al.*)
Class of evidence	II	II
Number of patients	170	216
Randomization	None	None
Follow-up	Lifetime of patients	Lifetime of patients
	Primary endpoint:	Primary endpoint:
	Survival	Survival
Stratification/ adjustments	Age	Age
	KPS	KPS
	Tumour histological subtype	Tumour histological subtype
	Tumour size	Tumour size
	Primary versus revision surgery	Tumour location

- Both studies used MRI to assess the extent of resection.
- The Baltimore group classified extent of resection according to the extent of fluid-attenuated inversion recovery (FLAIR) signal abnormality on MRI carried out <48 h post-operatively and classified EOR as follow: gross total resection (GTR); near total resection (NTR); and sub-total resection (STR).
- The San Francsico group calculated the percentage EOR using volumetric analysis of immediate post-operative MRI FLAIR signal on axial slices.

Outcomes

Survival was assessed by both groups and both groups used overall survival (OS) and progression-free survival (PFS) as outcome measures. Both studies also analysed survival without malignant progression of the tumour, with progression being defined as either radiological evidence (gadolinium-enhancement) or histological evidence of higher-grade tumour. Although slightly different terms were used by the two groups for malignant progression, for the sake of clarity this outcome will be defined here as malignant-free survival (MFS).

Results

Baltimore group (McGirt *et al.*)

	Gross total resection	Sub-total resection	Statistical significance
OS	15 years	9.9 years	$p = 0.017$
MFS	12.5 years	7.0 years	$p > 0.05$
PFS	7.0 years	3.5 years	$p = 0.043$

- GTR versus STR was associated with OS and PFS as shown in the table.
- There was no significant difference in survival rates between STR and NTR.

San Francisco group (Smith *et al.*)

	5-year survival		8-year survival	
	>90% resection	<90% resection	>90% resection	90% resection
OS	97%	76%	91%	60%
MFS	93%	72%	76%	48%
PFS	75%	40%	43%	21%

	Prognositc significance of EOR as a hazard ratio	Statistical significance
OS	0.972	$p < 0.001$
MFS	0.983	$p = 0.005$
PFS	0.992	$p > 0.05$

Conclusions

Baltimore group (McGirt *et al.*)

Greater EOR improves outcome for patients with LGG and should be safely attempted when not limited by eloquent cortex.

San Francisco group (Smith *et al.*)

Greater EOR improves outcome for adults patients with LGG.

Critique

Low-grade gliomas pose a particularly difficult management dilemma for neurosurgeons. The prognosis of LGGs can be up to ten-fold better than for high-grade gliomas. Although little is known about prognostic factors in these patients, the EOR has long been suspected to affect survival and early retrospective surgical series have been extremely influential in supporting this view (Laws *et al.*, 1984). There are no clinical trials specifically examining this question and meta-analysis of the literature would simply be a pooling of retrospective studies with widely varying statistical methodologies applied. Also, many earlier case series include histological grades that have now been better differentiated with more known about the influence of histological subtype on survival.

The question of whether extent of resection affects survival in LGG patients remains of utmost importance. LGGs are often in or near eloquent cortical regions and the risk of incurring neurological defects needs to be balanced against the need for total resection. With the more widespread application of neuronavigation and intra-operative MRI there is the possibility to perform more aggressive resections safely.

The two studies carried out here have their limitations which are acknowledged by the authors. Both studies are retrospective and do not include any comparisons with patients undergoing biopsy. Furthermore, there is the possibility that patients who underwent less than total resection may reflect cases where tumour had infiltrated so as to prevent safe resection and, therefore, were already likely to have a worse prognosis. Furthermore, there are potential methodological difficulties in using contrast enhancement as a measure of resection and of tumour progression. Notwithstanding these criticisms, these studies are perhaps the best studies to date that address the role of the extent of resection of low-grade gliomas on patient outcome.

A clinical trial addressing the role of EOR for LGG is unlikely to be forthcoming because of a lack of equipoise amongst neurosurgeons and potential difficulties recruiting enough patients due to the unwillingness of many patients to be randomized to the 'no resection' or 'biopsy only' arms (Smith *et al.*, 2008). The two retrospective series included here are landmark in that they are, and will continue to be, influential in guiding neuro-surgical decision-making regarding the EOR for LGG. It is likely that prospective studies evaluating the role of modalities such as intra-operative MRI will also be influential in guiding decision-making regarding the EOR. Indeed, there are already studies that suggest that using intra-operative MRI to help achieve total resection of LGG may improve survival when compared to known survival rates from national databases (Claus *et al.*, 2005).

Claus EB, Horlacher A, Hsu L, Schwartz RB, Dello-Iacono D, Talos F, Jolesz FA, Black PM. Survival rate in patients with low-grade glioma after intraoperative magnetic resonance image guidance. *Cancer* 2005; **103**: 1227–1233.

Laws ER Jr, Taylor WF, Clifton MB, Okazaki H. Neurosurgical management of low-grade astrocytoma of the cerebral hemispheres. *J Neurosurg* 1984; **61**: 66–673.

Smith JS, Chang EF, Lamborn KR, Chang SM, Prados MD, Cha S, Tihan T, Vandenberg S. Role of extent of resection in the long-term outcome of low-grade hemispheric gliomas. *J Clin Oncol* 2008; **10**: 1338–1345.

2.10 **Radiotherapy for low-grade gliomas**

Details of studies

There have been several trials evaluating the role of radiotherapy in the management of low-grade gliomas. These trials have been carried out in Europe by the European Organisation for Research and Treatment of Cancer (EORTC) and in North America by the North Center Cancer Treatment Group (NCCTG) in conjunction with the RTOG and the Eastern Cooperative Oncology Group (ECOG). The question of a dose–response relation for low-grade gliomas treated with radiotherapy was addressed by the first European Trial (EORTC I, or 'the believers trial') and the NCCTG-RTOG-ECOG trial ('the US trial'). The second European trial addressed the question of early versus delayed radiotherapy (at the time of disease progression) in low-grade glioma. These studies are, therefore, outlined below according to these two questions: low-dose versus high-dose radiotherapy; early versus delayed radiotherapy.

Study references

Main studies

EORTC I: 'Believers trial'

Karim AB, Maat B, Hatlevoll R, Menten J, Rutten EH, Thomas DG, Mascarenhas F, Horiot JC, Parvinen LM, van Reijn M, Jager JJ, Fabrini MG, van Alphen AM, Hamers HP, Gaspar L, Noordman E, Pierart M, van Glabbeke M. A randomized trial on dose-response in radiation therapy of low-grade cerebral glioma. European Organization for Research and Treatment of Cancer (EORTC) Study 22844. *Int J Rad Oncol Biol Phys* 1996; **36**: 549–556.

EORTC II: 'Non-believers trial'

Karim AB, Afra D, Cornu P, Bleehen N, Schraub S, De Witte O, Darcel F, Stenning S, Pierart M, Van Glabbeke M. Randomised trial on the efficacy of radiotherapy for cerebral low-grade glioma in the adult: European Organization for Research and Treatment of Cancer Study 22844 with the Medical Research Council study BRO4: an interim analysis. *Int J Rad Oncol Biol Phys* 2002; **52**: 316–324.

van den Bent MJ, Afra D, de Witte O, Ben Hassel M, Schraub S, Hoang-Xuan K, Malmström PO, Collette L, Piérart M, Mirimanoff R, Karim AB. EORTC Radiotherapy and Brain Tumor Groups and the UK Medical Research Council. Long-term efficacy of early versus delayed radiotherapy for low-grade astrocytoma and oligodendroglioma in adults: the EORTC 22845 randomised trial. *Lancet* 2005; **366**: 985–990.

NCCTG-RTOG-ECOG: 'US trial'

Shaw E, Arusell R, Scheithauer B, O'Fallon J, O'Neill B, Dinapoli R, Nelson D, Earle J, Jones C, Cascino T, Nichols D, Ivnik R, Hellman R, Curran W, Abrams R. Prospective randomized trial of low- versus high-dose radiation therapy in adults with supratentorial low-grade glioma: initial report of a North Central Cancer Treatment Group/Radiation Therapy Oncology Group/Eastern Cooperative Oncology Group Study. *J Clin Oncol* 2002; **20**: 2267–2276.

Related reference

Brown PD, Buckner JC, O'Fallon JR, Iturria NL, Brown CA, O'Neill BP, Scheithauer BW, Dinapoli RP, Arussel RM, Abrams RA, Curran WJ, Shaw EG. Adult patients with supratentorial pilocytic astrocytomas: a prospective multicenter clinical trial. *Int J Radiation Oncology Biol Phys* 2004; **58**: 1153–1160.

Study designs

+ All multi-centre PRCT

	Low-dose versus high-dose DXT		Early versus delayed DXT
	EORTC I 'Believers trial'	NCCTG-RTOG-ECOG 'US trial'	EORTC II 'Non-believers trial'
Class of evidence	I	I	I
Randomization	Low-dose versus high-dose DXT	Low-dose versus high-dose DXT	Early versus delayed DXT
Number of patients	379	203	311
Follow-up	≥50 months	15 years	Life span of patients (Minimum 60 months)
	Primary endpoints: Overall survival Progression of tumour	Primary endpoints: Overall survival Progression of tumour	Primary endpoints: Overall survival Progression of tumour
	Other endpoints: None	Other endpoints: Neurological status Cognitive function Toxicities	Other endpoints: Neurological status Cognitive function Seizures
	91% follow-up	100% follow-up	93% follow-up
Number of centres	27 centres in 10 countries	Unknown, but multiple	24
Stratification	Tumour grade Histological type Age Extent of resection	Tumour grade Histological type Age Extent of resection	Tumour grade Histological type Age Extent of resection

EORTC I ('believers trial')

+ Inclusion criteria: Adults (16–65 years); histological diagnosis of GI or GII supratentorial glioma (astrocytoma, oligodendroglioma, mixed oligodendroglioma).
+ Exclusion criteria: Poor neurological status; totally excised GI astrocytomas; pregnant patients; other 'incurable' malignancy.
+ DXT doses: Low (45 Gy); high (59.4 Gy).

NCCTG-RTOG-ECOG: The 'US trial'

+ Inclusion criteria: Adults (>18 years); histological diagnosis of supratentorial glioma (astrocytoma, oligodendroglioma, mixed oligoastrocytoma).
+ DXT doses: Low (50.4 Gy); high (64.8 Gy).

EORTC II: 'Non-believers trial'

- Inclusion criteria: Histological diagnosis of supratentorial low-grade glioma (GI/II astrocytoma; oligodendroglioma); KPS ≥60; adults (16–65 years).
- Exclusion criteria: Completely resected GI pilocytic astrocytoma; significant other malignancy; pregnancy.
- Dose of DXT: 54 Gy.
- Timing of DXT: Early (<8 weeks from surgery); delayed (at time of progression).
- Intention-to-treat analysis.

Outcome measures

EORTC I 'The believers trial'	NCCTG I 'The US trial'	EORTC II 'The non-believers trial'
Overall survival (OS) Progression-free survival at 5 years (PFS)	Overall survival (OS) Time to progression (TTP) Cognitive function: MMSE	Overall survival (OS) Time to progression (TTP) Cognitive function: MMSE

Results

Low-dose versus high-dose DXT

	EORTC I 'Believers trial'			NCCTG-RTOG-ECOG 'US trial'		
	Low-dose DXT	High-dose DXT	Statistical significance	Low-dose DXT	High-dose DXT	Statistical significance
5-Year survival	58%	59%	None	72%	65%	None
Progression (5-year PFS)	47%	50%	None	52%	50%	None

- In the 'believers trial', the following factors were significantly associated with better overall survival: Histology and grade (Grade I astrocytoma, oligodendroglioma, mixed oligodendroglioma); younger age.
- In the 'US trial', the following three factors were significantly associated with better overall survival: Histology (oligodendroglioma or oligo-dominant mixed tumours); young patients (<40 years); and smaller tumours (<5 cm).
- In the 'US trial', the combination of histology and age together was the most powerful prognostic indicator of 5-year survival: Patients with oligodendroglioma and <40 years (82%) versus patients with astrocytoma ≥40 years (32%).

Early versus delayed DXT

	Early DXT	Delayed DXT	Statistical significance
5-Year survival	63%	66%	None
5-Year PFS	44%	37%	$p = 0.02$

- There was no significant difference in the median survival for the early-DXT group (7.2 years) compared to the delayed-DXT group (7.4 years).
- However, patients in the delayed-DXT group survived significantly longer after progression than those in the early-DXT group (3.4 years versus 1.0 years, $p < 0.0001$).
- Post-hoc analysis revealed that significantly less patients in the early-DXT group suffered seizures in the first year (25% versus 41%).

Conclusions

- There is no improvement in survival with higher-dose radiotherapy ('believers trial' and 'US trial').
- Early radiotherapy does not improve overall survival, but it does lengthen progression-free survival ('non-believers trial').

Critique

Low-grade gliomas constitute approximately 10% of primary CNS malignancy, affect predominantly young adults, and are associated with a survival rates of <35% at 10 years. These trials have addressed two important questions regarding the role of radiotherapy to control this disease:

1 Is the effect of radiotherapy dose-dependent?

2 Is it better to administer radiotherapy early on or to delay administration until the disease progresses?

The EORTC I and NCCTG-RTOG-ECOG trials appear to support the use of lower-dose radiotherapy regimens. However, some feel that these trials cannot be interpreted clearly due to the histological heterogeneity of the gliomas included (Wessels *et al.*, 2003). One of the major weaknesses of the EORTC II study ('non-believers') is that the cohort includes both low- and high-grade gliomas as 26% of the tumours were reclassified as high-grade astrocytomas on histological review. In addition, over one-third of patients in the delayed-DXT group did not receive radiotherapy. It is felt by some that the fact that median survival was much greater following progression in the delayed-DXT group (2.4 years longer) could influence the decision when to give delayed-DXT (Knisely, 2006). The authors of the EORTC II study acknowledged that there was a lack of quality of life data, which would have allowed more considered discussion of their results.

The issues of dose–response and timing of radiotherapy in the management of low-grade gliomas remain controversial despite the results of these trials. Indeed,

Papagikos *et al.* have warned against an overly dogmatic approach to therapeutic options of low-grade gliomas in light of the conclusions from these trials (Papagikos *et al.*, 2005). There is considerable interest regarding the role of radiosurgery and adjuvant chemotherapy. A trial of radiotherapy versus radiotherapy plus chemotherapy was completed in the early 1990s, which did not show any benefit of adjuvant chemotherapy (Eyre *et al.*, 1993). However, new chemotherapeutic regimes are now being explored, which are tailored to specific histological types (Stege *et al.*, 2005; Wen and DeAngelis, 2007). The management of low-grade gliomas remains still predominantly in the domain of the specialist neuro-oncological surgeon and neuro-oncologist.

Eyre HJ, Crowley JJ, Townsend JJ, Eltringham JR, Morantz RA, Schulman SF, Quagliana JM, al-Samaf M. A randomised trial of radiotherapy versus radiotherapy plus CCNU for incompletely resected low-grade gliomas: a Southwest Oncology Group study. *J Neurosurg* 1993; **78**: 909–914.

Knisely J. Early or delayed radiotherapy for low-grade glioma? *Lancet Oncol* 2006; **6**: 921.

Papagikos MA, Shaw EG, Stieber VW. Lessons learned from randomised clinical trials in adult low-grade glioma. *Lancet Oncol* 2005; **6**: 240–244.

Stege EM, Kros JM, de Bruin HG, Enting RH, van Heuvel I, Looijenga LH, van der Rijt CD, Smitt PA, van den Bent MJ. Successful treatment of low-grade oligodendroglial tumors with a chemotherapy regimen of procarbazine, lomustine, and vincristine. *Cancer* 2005; **103**: 802–809.

Wen PY, DeAngelis LM. Chemotherapy for low-grade gliomas: emerging consensus on its benefits. *Neurology* 2007; **68**: 1762–1733.

Wessels PH, Weber WEJ, Raven G, Ramaekers FCS, Hopman AHN, Twijnstra A. Supratentorial grade II astroctyoma: biological features and clinical course. *Lancet Neurol* 2003; **2**: 395–402.

Chapter 3

Head injury

RD Johnson, T Santarius, JE Wilberger

3.0 **Introduction**

Head injuries are common, and moderate to severe traumatic brain injury (TBI) affects young and old alike with potentially high morbidity and mortality. Surgical treatment of head injury may represent the oldest neurosurgical procedures. Indeed, surgical options for head injuries are mentioned in the Edwin Smith papyrus, which refers to a period before 2500 BC (Breasted, 1930). In the modern era, neurosurgeons and neuro-intensivists are the main carers for this group of patients. Several advances have been influential in shaping current methods of management of head-injured patients. The pathologic nature of head injury has been further elucidated (Graham and Adams, 1971). As it appears that there is nothing that can be done to reverse the primary brain injury, the focus of our efforts is primarily targeted at the cascade of events leading to secondary brain injury. Efforts are directed at controlling intracranial pressure and maintaining adequate brain oxygenation and perfusion. This has required an increased cooperation between neuro-surgeons and neuro-intensivists. Another advance that has had a seismic impact in the early diagnosis of traumatic pathology in head-injured patients is the advent of cross-sectional computed tomography (CT) scanning (Hounsfield, 1973; French and Dublin, 1977): an advance that was recognized by the award of the 1979 Nobel Prize in medicine to Cormack and Hounsfield.

Mortality from civilian head injuries has been significantly reduced over the last 35 years (Seelig *et al.*, 1981). Nonetheless, many patients are left with extreme disabilities if they survive. The organization of head injury pharmacologic trials to improve outcome has been extremely difficult for logistical reasons and because of technical difficulties with their design (Narayan *et al.*, 2002). Dickinson *et al.* carried out a broad-range analysis of head injury trials, and in their analysis they reported several significant and dramatic findings (Dickinson *et al.*, 2000). First, they found that in the period up until 1998 there were a total of 208 discrete published randomized trials of interventions in head injury, but only 4% of these trials were of sufficient power to detect a 10% difference in outcome among the cohorts (power level set at 80%, $\beta = 0.2$). Second, they found that there were problems with blinding, not only in terms of patients and surgeons/doctors, but also of those evaluating outcome, with just over 20% of published trials with any blinding of outcome assessment. Dickinson *et al.* highlighted the small size of head injury trials, and calculated that the total number of patients enrolled in all head injury trials together up until 1998 was less than some of the larger individual trials in stroke and heart disease. A further consideration is that head injury is a heterogeneous group of entities and current classification systems, including those based on Glasgow Coma Scores (GCS), do not necessarily reflect this. It may be difficult, therefore, to derive useful information from head injury studies unless a large number of subjects have been included, and negative results from small studies should be treated with caution (Saatman *et al.*, 2008).

Several topics have been chosen for inclusion in this chapter that we feel are particularly relevant to the practising neurosurgeon and have addressed areas where there was sig-nificant equipoise. The opening section considers the landmark papers describing the Glasgow Coma Scale and Glasgow Outcome Scale that have had such a profound impact on the development and practice of neurosurgery (Teasdale and Jennett, 1974; Jennett and Bond, 1975). The next section deals with three seminal case studies regarding the timing of operative management of acute extradural and subdural haematomas (Mendelow *et al.*, 1979; Seelig *et al.*, 1981; Wilberger *et al.*, 1991). This is followed by a section that contains two studies addressing surgical technique for the management of chronic subdural haematomas (Svien and Gelety, 1964; Santarius *et al.*, 2009). Studies addressing the role of pharmacological interventions including steroids, barbiturates, hyperosmolar therapies, and magnesium have been included. Key studies addressing the efficacy of hypothermia have also been included. We have refrained from including any studies on the role of decompressive craniectomy in the management of adult head injury. This is primarily because the Randomized Evaluation of Surgery with Craniectomy for Uncontrollable Elevation of Intracranial Pressure (RESCUE-ICP) Study is still ongoing (Hutchinson *et al.*, 2006). In addition, a Cochrane review in 2006 concluded that there was no evidence to support the routine use of secondary decompressive craniectomy to reduce unfavourable outcome in adults with severe traumatic brain injury and refractory high ICPs (Sahuquillo and Arikan, 2006). There was, however, a suggestion from the results of non-randomized trials and controlled trials with historical controls that such surgery may be beneficial if maximal medical treatment fails to control intracranial pressure. The RESCUE-ICP and Early Decompressive Craniectomy in Patients with Severe Traumatic Brain Injury (DECRA) studies are currently ongoing to test the hypothesis that decompressive craniectomy in head-injured patients with raised and refractory ICP results in improvement in outcome compared to optimal medical management. The next section looks at a seminal study that addressed the role of hyperventilation on outcome in head injury (Muizelaar *et al.*, 1991). The final two sections of this chapter address landmark studies in post-traumatic seizures (PTS) following head injury. The penultimate section considers a population-based study of PTS by Annegers *et al.* (1998), which is the largest of its kind taking in 4541 patients over a period of 50 years and has produced the most accurate data regarding the epidemiology of PTS. The study emphasizes the importance of this problem with 2–4 people per 100,000 suffering from a severe traumatic head injury each year with an incidence of PTS in 30% or over these patients. The final section addresses a randomized, double-blind trial of phenytoin for the prophylaxis of PTS (Temkin *et al.*, 1990). Although many studies had already been published on seizure prophylaxis for post-traumatic epilepsy, Temkin's study stands out as being the largest study with sufficient power to be able to analyse the efficacy of phenytoin. The results of Temkin's study have been confirmed by several meta-analyses of all published trials.

This chapter refers almost exclusively to the adult population. Two further studies looking at the issues of decompressive craniectomy and hypothermia in paediatric head injury have been included in the paediatric neurosurgery chapter. Furthermore, the head injury guidelines drawn up by the United States Brain Trauma Foundation are based on their Task Force review of the available evidence (Bullock *et al.*, 2006; Brain Trauma Foundation, 2007). These guidelines are a landmark in neurosurgery and are recommended reading for all those with an interest in head injury.

Annegers JF, Hauser WA, Coan SP, Rocca WA. A population-based study of seizures after traumatic brain injuries. *N Engl J Med* 1998; **338**: 20–24.

Brain Trauma Foundation – Bullock MR, Povlishock (Eds). Guidelines for the management of severe traumatic brain injury. *J Neurotrauma* 2007; **24**: S1–S106.

Breasted JH. The Edwin Smith surgical papyrus. (Chicago, 1930) University of Chicago Press.

Bullock MR, Chestnut R, Ghajar J, Gordon D, Hartl R, Newell DW, Servadei F, Walters BC, Wilberger JE. Surgical management of TBI author group. *Neurosurgery* 2006; **58**: S2-1–S2-3.

Dickinson K, Bunn F, Wentz R, Edwards P, Roberts I. Size and quality of randomised controlled trials in head injury: review of published studies. *BMJ* 2000; **320**: 1308–1311.

French BN, Dublin AB. The value of computerized tomography in the management of 1000 consecutive head injuries. *Surg Neurol* 1977; **7**: 171–183.

Hounsfield GN. Computerized transverse axial scanning (tomography). 1. Description of system. *Br J Radiol* 1973; **46**: 1016–1022.

Hutchinson PJ, Corteen E, Czosnyka M, Mendelow AD, Menon DK, Mitchell P, Murray G, Pickard JD, Rickels E, Sahuquillo J, Servadei F, Teasdale GM, Timofeev I, Unterberg A, Kirkpatrick PJ. Decompressive craniectomy in traumatic brain injury: the randomized multicenter RESCUEicp study (www.RESCUEicp.com). *Acta Neurochir Suppl* 2006; **96**: 17–20.

Jennett B, Bond M. Assessment of outcome after severe brain damage: a practical scale. *Lancet* 1975; **1**: 480–484.

Mendelow AD, Karmi MZ, Paul KS, Fuller GAG, Gillingham FJ. Extradural haematomas: effect of delayed treatment. *Br Med J* 1979; **1**: 1240–1249.

Muizelaar JP, Marmarou A, Ward JD, Kontos HA, Choi SC, Becker DP, Gruemer H, Young HF. Adverse effects of prolonged hyperventilation in patients with severe traumatic brain injury. *J Neurosurg* 1991; **75**: 731–739.

Narayan RK, Michel ME, Ansell B, Baethmann A, Biegon A, Bracken MB, Bullock MR, Choi SC, Clifton GL, Contant CF, Coplin WM, Dietrich WD, Ghajar J, Grady SM, Grossman RG, Hall ED, Heetderks W, Hovda DA, Jallo J, Katz RL, Knoller N, Kochanek PM, Maas AI, Majde J, Marion DW, Marmarou A, Marshall LF, McIntosh TK, Miller E, Mohberg N, Muizelaar JP, Pitts LH, Quinn P, Riesenfeld G, Robertson CS, Strauss KI, Teasdale G, Temkin N, Tuma R, Wade C, Walker MD, Weinrich M, Whyte J, Wilberger JE, Young AB, Yurkewicz L. Clinical trials in head injury. *J Neurotrauma* 2002; **19**: 503–557.

Saatman KE, Duhaime AC, Bullock R, Maas AI, Valadka A, Manley GT; Workshop Scientific Team and Advisory Panel Members. Classification of traumatic brain injury for targeted therapies. *J Neurotrauma* 2008; **25**: 719–738.

Sahuquillo J, Arikan F. Decompressive craniectomy for the treatment of refractory high intracranial pressure in traumatic brain injury. *Cochrane Database Syst Rev* 2006; 1:CD003983.

Santarius T, Kirkpatrick PJ, Ganesan D, Chia HL, Jallah I, Smielewski P, Richards HK, Marcus H, Parker RA, Price SH, Kirollos RW, Pickard JD, Hutchinson PJ. Use of drains versus no drains after burr-hole evacuation of chronic subdural haematoma: a randomised controlled trial. *Lancet* 2009; **374**: 1067–1073.

Seelig JM, Becker DP, Miller JD, *et al*. Traumatic acute subdural hematoma: major mortality reduction in comatose patients treated within four hours. *JAMA* 1981; **304**: 1511–1518.

Svien HJ, Gelety JE. On the surgical management of encapsulated subdural hematoma. *J Neurosurgery* 1964; **21**: 172–177.

Teasdale G, Jennett B. Assessment of coma and impaired consciousness: a practical scale. *Lancet* 1974; **2**: 81–84.

Temkin NR, Dikmen SS, Wilensky AJ, Keihm J, Chabal S, Winn HR. A randomised, double-blind study of phenytoin for the prevention of post-traumatic seizures. *N Engl J Med* 1990; **323**: 497–502.

Wilberger JE, Harris M, Diamond DL. Acute sudbural haematoma: morbidity, mortality and operative timing. *J Neurosurg* 1991; **74**: 212–218.

3.1 **Glasgow Coma Scale and Glasgow Outcome Scale**

Details of studies

Teasdale and Jennett first described the Glasgow Coma Scale (GCS) in 1974 (Teasdale and Jennett, 1974). The GCS has become the most widely used scoring system for describing the neurologic status in head-injured patients worldwide. The Glasgow Outcome Scale (GOS) was first reported by Jennett and Bond in 1975 (Jennett and Bond, 1975). The GCS and GOS have become a widely accepted method of reporting outcomes not only in studies of head injuries, but also in other neurosurgical conditions.

Study references

Main studies

Jennett B, Bond M. Assessment of outcome after severe brain damage. *Lancet* 1975; **1**: 480–484.

Jennett B, Snoek J, Bond MR, Brooks N. Disability after severe head injury: observations on the use of the Glasgow Outcome Scale. *J Neurol Neurosurg Psychiatr* 1981; **44**: 285–293.

Teasdale G, Jennett B. Assessment of coma and impaired consciousness. A practical scale. *Lancet* 1974; **2**: 81–84.

Teasdale G, Jennett B. Assessment and prognosis of coma after head injury. *Acta Neurochir* 1976; **34**: 45–55.

Related references

Jennett B, Teasdale G. Aspects of coma after severe head injury. *Lancet* 1977; 878–881.

Jennett B, Teasdale G, Galbraith S, Pickard J, Grant H, Braakman R, Avezaat C, Mass A, Minderhoud J, Vecht C, Heiden J, Small R, Caten W, Kurze T. Severe head injuries in three countries. *J Neurol Neurosurg Pyschiatr* 1977; **40**: 291–298.

Glasgow Coma Scale

The original GCS was described as follows:

> A clinical scale has been evolved for assessing the depth and duration of impaired consciousness and coma. Three aspects of behaviour are independently measured – motor responsiveness, verbal performance, and eye opening.
>
> Jennett and Teasdale (1974)

The first description in 1974 consisted of a 14-point scale as follows:

Eye opening	Best verbal response	Best motor response
Spontaneous	Orientated	Obeying
To speech	Confused	Localizing
To pain	Inappropriate	Flexing
None	Incomprehensible	Extending
	None	None

However, numerical values were not added until it was modified to a 15-point scale in 1976:

Eye opening		Best verbal response		Best motor response	
Response	Score	Response	Score	Response	Score
Spontaneous	4	Orientated	5	Obeying	6
To speech	3	Confused	4	Localizing	5
To pain	2	Inappropriate	3	Withdrawing	4
None	1	Incomprehensible	2	Flexing	3
		None	1	Extending	2
				None	1

The assessment of motor response was described in detail with 'obeying commands' being defined as the best response possible. Jennett and Teasdale emphasized that this response should be interpreted carefully:

> The observer must take care not to interpret a grasp reflex or a postural adjustment as a response to command. The terms 'purposeful' and 'voluntary' are avoided as we believe they cannot be judged objectively.
>
> Jennett and Teasdale (1974)

The authors also described in detail the method by which noxious stimuli were to be applied starting with pressure on the nail bed with a pencil to test for flexion and then to the head, neck, or trunk to test for localization. Motor responses are described in detail: localizing is defined as a limb moving to remove a noxious stimulus at more than one site (e.g. the opposite limb moving to site of nail bed pressure); withdrawing is normal flexion of the elbow or knee to local painful stimulus; abnormal flexion is slow withdrawal with pronation of the wrist and adduction of the shoulder; extensor response is defined as adduction and internal rotation of the shoulder with pronation of the forearm. They also indicate the importance of recording the best motor response if there is a discrepancy between limbs as the lesser response may reflect localized brain damage rather than over-all conscious level. They indicate that eye opening in response to pain should be assessed from stimulus to the limbs to avoid the grimacing reflex causing eye closure. Verbal responses are described as follows: orientated (in time, place, person); confused conversation (attends and responds to questions but with incorrect or muddled answers); inappropriate words (intelligible words but random and unrelated to questions asked); incomprehensible speech (moans and groans only).

Glasgow Outcome Scale

The original GOS described in 1975 had included four categories of survivors and one category for death as follows:

Death	
Vegetative state	No evidence of meaningful response
Severe disability	Conscious but needs the assistance of another person for either physical or mental reasons
Moderate disability	Independent but disabled
Good recovery	Resumption of normal occupation and social activities

Patients in a vegetative state were said to be able to breathe spontaneously and may even eye open, swallow, or show reflex responses in the limbs. However, a vegetative state was said to indicate a lack of function of the cerebral cortex. The three categories of disability described a range of physical and mental dependencies. However, as it was felt that these categories were so compressed as to be insensitive to degrees of improvement within each category the scale was extended in 1981 to further subdivide each disability category into two subcategories (upper and lower) so that, including death as an outcome, an 8-point scale was produced.

Critique

The GCS is the most widely utilized scale for the measurement of level of consciousness worldwide. The GCS has been incorporated into other scores of ill health and trauma including the Acute Physiology and Chronic Health Evaluation (APACHE) II score and the Trauma and Injury Severity Score (TRISS). Indeed, the only country that has ever rejected the GCS in favour of another scoring system is Sweden (Starmark et al., 1988; Marion and Carlier, 1994). Despite its widespread acceptance and use, the GCS has not been without its critics. Although the GCS was developed primarily as a research tool in order to predict outcome and to allow for bedside assessments of fluctuations of conscious level, it has been widely utilized as an indicator for clinical decision-making. This is demonstrated by the adage 'If the GCS is less than 8, then you need to intubate'. The GCS score has become utilized to alert practitioners to the need to protect the airway with formal intubation (Chestnut, 1997). Likewise a GCS of 8 is a threshold for consideration of ICP monitoring. However, using the GCS in these ways implies that it is summarized as a single numerical score. Jennett and Teasdale assigned a numerical score to the GCS and in their assessment of 700 head-injured patients concluded that all combinations that resulted in a GCS of <8 were definitive of coma (Jennett and Teasdale, 1977). However, they have always emphasized that the conscious level of a patient should always be described fully in terms of the three separate responses (Teasdale et al., 1983). Indeed, the summation of the score to a single figure has been criticized for weighting the motor score over the other components (Bhatty and Kapoor, 1993). However, this weighting towards the motor score may be desirable as it is possible that the motor response is the best predictor of neurological outcome (Jagger et al., 1983). The other main criticism of the GCS is the fact that it does not incorporate any measure of brainstem reflexes (Segatore and Way, 1992). However, the original aim of the GCS was to produce a scale that provided interobserver reliability so that frequent and repeated assessments could be made by the bedside. Scoring systems that have incorporated brainstem reflexes have been more complicated and, therefore, less inter-rater reliability. Jennett and Teasdale made it clear in their original description that the GCS was not developed to replace a full neurological examination:

> It is no part of our case to deny the value of a detailed appraisal of the patient as a whole, and of neurological function in particular
>
> (Jennett and Teasdale, 1974)

Another area of criticism of the GCS is its application to intubated patients: a problem that is generally circumvented by recording the verbal score with a 'T' (Meredith *et al.*, 1988). Furthermore, there have been concerns regarding the use of the GCS in the pre-hospital setting as it appears that such scores may not correlate with either severity of head injury or serve as prognostic indicators of outcome (Marion and Carlier, 1994). Notwithstanding these weaknesses and criticisms, the description of the GGS was a true landmark in neurosurgery as it brought consistency to scoring conscious levels in head-injured patients and all the evidence indicates that it is likely to remain in widespread use for a long time to come.

The aim of the GOS was to describe overall social outcome in patients in terms of a limited set of outcomes, which were 'sufficiently clearly defined to be used reliably by observers in several centres, some of whom were in different countries' (Jennett *et al.*, 1981). Almost immediately after the GOS was described, it was proposed by others that it should be adopted worldwide for the follow-up of series of head-injured patients (Langfitt, 1978). The original GOS was, however, relatively insensitive to subtle changes and for weighting physical disability relative to cognitive dysfunction (Kaye and Andrews, 2000). It appears that most patients will reach their final point on the 5-point scale by 6 months: an interval at which it is also usually possible to successfully follow-up patients (Jennett, 2005). Indeed, it appears that early GOS at 3 months correlates well with long-term GOS (King *et al.*, 2005). Modification of the GOS to the Glasgow Outcome Score—Extended (GOS-E) has addressed this and the GOS-E has been found to be more sensitive for detecting changes in mild to moderate head-injured patients, particularly when assessed on the basis of a structured interview, and thus more useful for longer-term follow-up (Wilson *et al.*, 1998; Levin *et al.*, 2001). In many research papers, outcomes are dichot-omized into 'poor' (severe disability or vegetative state) or 'good' (moderate disability or good recovery).

The GCS and GOS have been widely adopted for the management and study of trau-matic and non-traumatic patients. Jennett has emphasized that training in their proper use is necessary to ensure that they are not misleading (Jennett, 2005).

Bhatty GB, Kapoor N. The Glasgow Coma Scale: a mathematical critique. *Acta Neurochir* 1993; **120**: 132–135.

Chestnut RM. The management of severe traumatic brain injury. *Emerg Med Clin North Am* 1997; **15**: 581–604.

Jagger J, Jane JA, Rimet R. The Glasgow Coma Scale: to sum or not to sum? [letter] *Lancet* 1983; **2**: 97.

Jennett B. Development of the Glasgow Coma and Outcome Scales. *Nepal J Neurosci* 2005; **2**: 24–28.

Kaye AH, Andrews D. Glasgow Outcome Scale: research scale or blunt instrument? *Lancet* 2000; **356**: 1540–1541.

King JT, Jr., Carlier PM, Marion DW. Early Glasgow Outcome Scale scores predict long-term functional outcome in patients with severe traumatic brain injury. *J Neurotrauma* 2005; **22**: 947–954.

Langfitt TW. Measuring the outcome from head injuries. *J Neurosurg* 1978; **48**: 673–678.

Levin HS, Boake C, Song J, McCauley S, Contant C, Diaz-Marchan P, Brundage S, Goodman H, Kotrla KJ. Validity and sensitivity to change of the extended Glasgow Outcome Scale in mild to moderate traumatic brain injury. *J Neurotrauma* 2001; **18**: 575–584.

Marion DW, Carlier PM. Problems with intitial Glasgow Coma Scale assessment caused by prehospital treatment of patients with head injuries: results of a national survery. *J Trauma* 1994; **36**: 89–95.

Meredith W, Rutledge R, Fakhry SM, Emery S, Kromhout-Schiro S. The conundrum of the Glasgow Coma Scale in intubated patients: a linear regression prediction of the Glasgow verbal score from the Glasgow eye and motor scores. *J Trauma* 1988; **44**: 839–845.

Segatore M, Way C. The Glasgow Coma Scale: time for a change. *Heart Lung* 1992; **21**: 548–557.

Starmark JE, Stålhammar D, Holmgren E, Rosander B. A comparison of the Glasgow Coma Scale and the Reaction Level Scale (RLS85). *J Neurosurg* 1988; **69**: 699–706.

Teasdale G, Jennett B, Murray L, Murray G. Glasgow Coma Scale: to sum or not to sum? [letter] *Lancet* 1983; **2**: 678.

Wilson JT, Pettigrew LE, Teasdale GM. Structured interviews for the Glasgow Outcome Scale and the Extended Glasgow Outcome Scale: guidelines for their use. *J Neurotrauma* 1998; **15**: 573–585.

3.2 **Timing of surgery for acute traumatic extra-axial haematomas**

Details of studies

Three seminal case series concerned with the timing of surgery to evacuate extra-axial haematomas are included in this section. The first is a series of 83 patients treated for traumatic extradural haematomas (EDH) in the Edinburgh area in the periods 1951–1960 and 1968–1977 (Mendelow *et al.*, 1979). This series compared the effects on outcome of delayed treatment following neurological deterioration and emphasized the need for immediate operation in patients deteriorating from extradural haematomas. The second study is a series of 82 patients with traumatic acute subdural haematomas (ASDH) admitted to the Division of Neurological Surgery, Medical College of Virginia between 1972 and 1980 (Seelig *et al.*, 1981). This paper established the principle of time to definitive surgical treatment as the most significant factor in the management of traumatic acute subdural haematomas. The third study is a series of 101 patients with traumatic ASDH admitted to Allegheny General Hospital between 1982 and 1987. This paper, while confirming the general trend regarding the effect of timing of surgery on outcome, highlighted the importance of control of ICP and the effect of primary brain injury.

Study references

Main studies

Mendelow AD, Karmi MZ, Paul KS, Fuller GAG, Gillingham FJ. Extradural haematomas: effect of delayed treatment. *Br Med J* 1979; **1**: 1240–1249.

Seelig JM, Becker DP, Miller JD, *et al.* Traumatic acute subdural hematoma: major mortality reduction in comatose patients treated within four hours. *JAMA* 1981; **304**: 1511–1518.

Wilberger JE, Harris M, Diamond DL. Acute sudbural haematoma: morbidity, mortality and operative timing. *J Neurosurg* 1991; **74**: 212–218.

Related reference

Bullock MR, Chestnut R, Ghajar J, Gordon D, Hartl R, Newell DW, Servadi F, Walters BC, Wilberger JE; Surical Management of Traumatic Brain Injury Author Group. Surgical management of acute subdural haematomas. *Neurosurgery* 2006; **58**: S16–S24.

Study designs

+ All retrospective case series

	Mendelow et al. (1979)	Seelig et al. (1981)	Wilberger et al. (1991)
Class of evidence	III	III	III
Number of patients	83	82	101
Number of centres	1 (Edingburgh, Scotland, UK)	1 (Richmond, Virginia, USA)	1 (Pittsburgh, Pensylvania, USA)
Outcomes	◆ Mortality ◆ Functional status	◆ Mortality ◆ Functional status (GOS)	◆ Mortality ◆ Functional status (GOS)
Eligibility	◆ Extradural haematoma >1.5 cm thick ◆ No depressed skull fracture present	◆ ASDH causing >5 mm midline shift ◆ Neurological status: impaired verbal response (unable to speak in response to noxious stimuli); unresponsive to verbal command ◆ Negative drug/alcohol screen ◆ Spontaneous respiration	◆ ASDH ◆ GCS <8 after resuscitation ◆ Absence of brain death ◆ No hypotensive episodes (<90 mmHg for >30 min) ◆ No other life threatening injuries ◆ Negative drug/alcohol screens
Treatment	◆ Surgical evacuation of clot	◆ Comprehensive resuscitation including the use of mannitol ◆ Rapid temporal craniectomy + partial clot evacuation followed by immediate temperofron-toparietal craniotomy. ◆ Contused/necrotic temporal and frontal brain removed where appropriate	◆ Comprehensive resuscitation including the use of mannitol ◆ Rapid craniotomy and removal of clot plus resection of any necrotic brain tissue and placement of intraventricular catheter

◆ In the study by Mendelow et al. delay was defined as the time between neurological deterioration and surgery.

◆ In the studies by Seelig et al. and Wilberger et al. delay was defined as time from injury to surgery.

Results

Mendelow et al. (1979)

In the study by Mendelow the two time periods compared reflected a change in the management of head-injured patients: in the second time period, patients were routinely admitted directly to the neurosurgical unit within 24 h. This resulted in a four-fold reduction in delay to surgery ($p = 0.06$).

Delay to surgery in survivors	Delay to surgery in non-survivors	Statistical significance
1.9 h	15.7 h	$p < 0.05$

Seelig et al. (1981)

	Surgery <4 h from injury	Surgery >4 h from injury	Statistical significance
Mortality	30%	90%	$p < 0.0001$

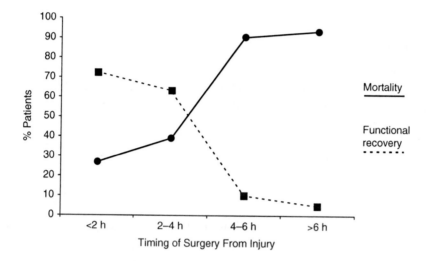

- Post-operative control of ICP <20 mmHg was associated with a functional recovery in 79% of patients ($p < 0.001$).

- Poor pre-operative neurological status was associated with an increased mortality ($p < 0.05$).

Wilberger et al. (1991)

- Although there was a trend for earlier surgery to improve mortality rates and functional recovery this was only statistically significant in patients who underwent surgery >12 h following injury ($p < 0.05$).

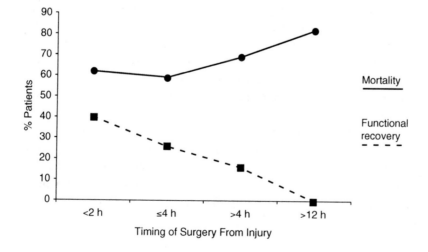

- Poor pre-operative neurological status (GCS <5) was significantly associated with high mortality (>75%, $p < 0.05$).
- Control of ICP was significantly associated with mortality and functional recovery: mortality with ICP <20 mmHg was 40% compared to a mortality of >95% with ICP >45 mmHg ($p < 0.05$); no patients with ICP >45 mmHg had a functional recovery ($p < 0.05$).

Conclusions

Mendelow et al. (1979)

- Delay in surgical evacuation of EDH leads to increased morbidity and mortality, with delays of more than 2 h being unacceptable.

Seelig et al. (1981)

- The diagnosis and surgical evacuation of ASDH within 4 h of injury considerably reduces mortality.

Wilberger et al. (1991)

- Although timely evacuation of ASDH is warranted, effective control of intracranial pressure appears to be more critical to outcome.

Critique

Extra-axial haematomas have long been considered surgically curable pathologic entities and it has long been recognized that evacuation at the earliest opportunity may be beneficial (Putnam and Cushing, 1925; Chambers, 1951). The study by Mendelow et al. supported this view in the case of extradural haematomas with their finding that the mean delay to surgery was more than 8 times longer in non-survivors (15.7 h) than survivors (1.9 h). The aim of the sudy by Mendelow was primarily to evaluate the effect of a change in head injury services in Edinburgh between two time periods. In the second time period, head-injured patients were admitted to a neurosurgical unit for 24 h routinely. This practice certainly reduced delays to surgery to a degree that almost reached statistical significance ($p = 0.06$). There have been other studies that have supported the immediate surgical intervention for EDH (Bricolo and Pasut, 1984). However, the series by Mendelow et al. is often cited as providing clear evidence that delay in evacuation following clinical deterioration is associated with worsening of outcome.

The series by Seelig et al. is a landmark in the field of head injury as it established the earliest possible evacuation of ASDH, and preferably within 4 h, as a benchmark of neurosurgical care. The later series by Wilberger et al., although broadly supporting this finding, also revealed that the extent of the underlying primary brain injury and appropriate strategies to prevent secondary brain injury may be more important than the timing of surgery in determining outcome. This study is also a landmark, particularly because it has led to an increased focus on how to manage ICP during the interval between injury and surgery.

These landmark studies that have been highly influential in establishing the general acceptance of timely intervention for traumatic extra-axial haematomas are the benchmark. Nonetheless, it should be recognized that there are studies that suggest there may be a role for a conservative approach in selected patients: in particular those with small-volume haematomas that do not cause compression or midline shift (Hamilton and Wallace, 1992; Croce et al., 1994; Servadi et al., 1998). Nonetheless, there is little contention regarding the role of emergency surgery in patients deteriorating from traumatic extra-axial lesions. Indeed, discussions regarding the evidence to support surgery in this situation have been likened to discussions about the evidence for the benefits for parachutes in determining outcome for sky-divers. However, there is an area of traumatic head injury that remains more controversial and that is the role of surgery in patients with traumatic contusions or traumatic intraparenchymal haematomas. In this setting, it appears that neurosurgeons are much more conservative in their approach and there appears to be enough equipoise to facilitate a large multi-centre randomized trial (Compagne et al., 2005). Indeed, the STITCH (trauma) trial started recruiting patients in 2009 (http://research.ncl.ac.uk/trauma.STITCH/).

Further developments have been made with regard to optimizing other variables such as pre-hospital resuscitation and control of cerebral perfusion and intracranial pressure. However, traumatic EDH and ASDH represent a diverse population of patients and comprehensive guidelines have been developed by leading expert groups on how to best manage these lesions (Bullock et al., 2006a; Bullock et al., 2006b).

Bricolo AP, Pasut LM. Extradural hematoma: toward zero mortality. A prospective study. *Neurosurgery* 1984; **14**: 8–12.

Bullock MR, Chestnut R, Ghajar J, Gordon D, Hartl R, Newell DW, Servadi F, Walters BC, Wilberger JE; Surgical Management of Traumatic Brain Injury Author Group. Surgical management of acute subdural haematomas. *Neurosurgery* 2006a; **58**: S7–S15.

Bullock MR, Chestnut R, Ghajar J, Gordon D, Hartl R, Newell DW, Servadi F, Walters BC, Wilberger JE; Surgical Management of Traumatic Brain Injury Author Group. Surgical management of acute subdural haematomas. *Neurosurgery* 2006b; **58**: S16–S24.

Chambers JW. Acute subdural hematoma. *J Neurosurg* 1951; **8**: 263–268.

Compagne C, Murray GD, Teasdale GM, Maas AIR, Esposito D, Princi P, D'Avella D, Servadi F. The management of patients with intradural post-traumatic mass lesions: a multi-centre survey of current approaches to surgical management in 729 patients coordinated by the European Brain Injury Consortium. *Neurosurgery* 2005; **57**: 1183–1191.

Croce MA, Dent DL, Menke PG, Robertson JT, Hinson MS, Young BH, Donovan TB, Pritchard FE, Minard G, Kudsk KA. Acute subdural haematoma: nonsurgical management of selected patients. *J Trauma* 1994; **36**: 820–826.

Hamilton M, Wallace C. Non-operative management of acute epidural hematoma diagnosed by CT: the neuroradiologist's role. *AJNR* 1992; **13**: 853–859.

Putnam TJ, Cushing H. Chronic subdural hematoma: its pathology, its relation to pachymeningitis hemorrhagia and its surgical treatment. *Arch Surg* 1925; **11**: 329–393.

Servadi F, Nasi MT, Cremoni AM, Giuliani G, Cenni P, Nanni A. Importance of a reliable admission Glasgow Coma Scale score for determining the need for evacuation of posttraumatic subdural hematomas: a prospective study of 65 patients. *J Trauma* 1998; **44**: 868–873.

3.3 Surgery for chronic subdural haematomas

Details of studies

Two studies are included in this section. First is a series of 69 patients with chronic subdural haematoma (CSDH) treated between 1955 and 1960 either with craniotomy or burr hole evacuation (Svien and Gelety, 1964). This was the first study to demonstrate that burr hole evacuation is an overall better operation than craniotomy for the treatment of primary CSDH. Second is a randomized controlled trial addressing one of the key questions regarding the surgical management of CSDH, namely the role of drains following burr hole evacuation (Santarius et al., 2009). The trial was carried out at Addenbrooke's Hospital in Cambridge between 2004 and 2007.

Study references

Main studies

Svien HJ and Gelety JE. On the surgical management of encapsulated subdural hematoma. *J Neurosurgery* 1964; **21**: 172–177.

Santarius T, Kirkpatrick PJ, Ganesan D, Chia HL, Jallah I, Smielewski P, Richards HK, Marcus H, Parker RA, Price SH, Kirollos RW, Pickard JD, Hutchinson PJ. Use of drains versus no drains after burr-hole evacuation of chronic subdural haematoma: a randomised controlled trial. *Lancet* 2009; **374**: 1067–1073.

Related references

Weigel R, Schmiedek P, Krauss JK. Outcome of contemporary surgery for chronic subdural haematoma: evidence based review. *J Neurol Neurosurg Psychiatry* 2003; **74**: 937–943.

Lega BC, Danish SF, Malhotra NR, Sonnad SS, Stein SC. Choosing the best operation for chronic subdural hematoma: a decision analysis. *J Neurosurg* 2009 October 30. Ahead of print.

Svien and Gelety, 1964

Study design

* Case series

Class of evidence	III
Comparing	Craniotomy versus burr hole evacuation
Number of patients	69
Outcomes	Recurrence requiring re-drainage Functional outcome at discharge Functional outcome at follow-up (3 months to 8 years)
Number of centres	1

* Inclusion criteria: Age >18 years; symptomatic CSDH confirmed on CT scan, presence of CSDH membranes confirmed pre-operatively.
* Exclusion criteria: Patients with radiological evidence of skull fracture, severe associated injuries or history of unconsciousness of more than 5 min.

Results

	Burr hole drainage	Craniotomy	Statistical significance*
Recurrence	10/50 (20%)	7/19(37%)	$p = 0.15\%$
Good functional status at discharge (%)†	98%	83%	$p = 0.065\%$

*Not done in the paper.

†Data on the functional status at follow-up are too complex for presentation in a table.

Conclusions

◆ Burr hole evacuation is a preferred technique to craniotomy in the treatment of CSDH.

Santarius *et al.*, 1968

Study design

◆ Randomized controlled trial

Class of evidence	I
Randomization	Drain versus no drain
Number of patients	215
Follow-up	Primary outcomes: Recurrence requiring re-drainage
	Secondary outcomes: Mortality at 30 days and 6 months
	100% follow-up for primary outcome and 98% for secondary outcomes
Number of centres	1

◆ Inclusion criteria: Age >18 years; symptomatic CSDH confirmed on CT scan.

◆ Exclusion criteria: Indication for surgery other than burr hole evacuation; insertion of CSF shunt ipsilateral to CSDH within preceding 6 months; use of drain deemed unsafe by surgeon.

◆ Analysis was carried out on an intention-to-treat basis.

Results

	Drain	No drain	Statistical significance
Recurrence	9.3%	24%	$p = 0.003\%$
Mortality at 6 months	8.6%	18.1%	$p = 0.042\%$

◆ The trial was stopped early because of the significant benefit in reduction of recurrence with the use of a drain.

◆ At discharge, patients with drains were reported to have fewer neurological deficits, a better functional status, and more favourable modified Rankin scores.

- There were no significant differences in complication rates between the two groups.

Conclusions

- Use of a drain following burr hole drainage of chronic subdural haematoma is safe and associated with reduced recurrence and mortality at 6 months.

Critique

CSDH is common clinical problem associated with considerable morbidity and mortality. There are numerous surgical options available to address this problem and an equally large number of opinions in the neurosurgical field as to which is the best technique. In this section we discuss two papers. The first has initiated a change in practice from that of craniotomy to burr hole drainage being the treatment of choice for primary CSDH. The second has provided randomized trial level of evidence for the use of drains with burr hole drainage and is likely to change practice from not using to using drains.

Until the paper by Svien and Gelety, the prevailing method of treatment of CSDH, including primary CSDH, was craniotomy (Markwalder, 1981; Markwalder and Seiler, 1985; Hamilton *et al.*, 1993). The authors showed, for the first time, that it is not necessary to perform craniotomy and membranectomy for CSDH. In fact, the outcome was better and the recurrence rate lower, although the latter not reaching statistical significance. The standard of the evidence presented in this paper is barely of Class III, and a lot of criticism can be made about the rigorousness of the definition of clinical status of patents at discharge and follow-up. However, following this study, numerous prospective and retrospective case series as well as two meta-analyses have confirmed findings of the paper by Svien and Gelety (Weigel *et al.*, 2003; Lega *et al.*, 2009; Mondorf *et al.*, 2009).

As many surgeons prefer minicraniotomies as the method of choice for evacuation of CSDH, believing that these are associated with lower recurrence rate, it would be beneficial to compare these two techniques in a clinical trial (Hamilton *et al.*, 1993; Lee *et al.*, 2009; Mondorf *et al.*, 2009).

In addition to the discussion of craniotomy versus burr hole craniostomy, there has been an ongoing debate about the merits of drains with burr hole craniostomy. Therefore, in their trial, Santarius *et al.* have chosen to examine a single question: Does the use of a drain when carrying out burr hole craniostomy for CSDH affect outcome? The authors concede that their trial has the weakness of being a single-centre study. However, the trial has certainly been successful in answering the question it addressed and the results are consistent with previous prospective studies (Wakai *et al.*, 1990; Tsutsumi *et al.*, 1997).

There has also been reluctance among some neurosurgeons to use drains because of concerns about potential complications of drain insertion. However, this trial by Santarius *et al.*, similarly to other studies, did not find any significant difference in complication rates with the use of a drain (Mori and Maeda, 2001; Lind *et al.*, 2003).

This trial stands out as a landmark study by showing that a simple additional intervention can have a significant beneficial effect on patient outcome. This finding was in marked contrast to the widely held beliefs regarding the use of drains (Santarius *et al.*, 2008).

This trial has also opened the way for further trials to evaluate important questions in the management of chronic subdural haematomas. Is there a role for steroids to prevent recurrence, for example? Undoubtedly, there will be further trials comparing operative techniques and perhaps even larger mutli-centre trials.

Hamilton MG, Frizzell JB, Tranmer BI. Chronic subdural hematoma: the role for craniotomy reevaluated. *Neurosurgery* 1993; **33**: 67–72.

Lee JK, Choi JH, Kim CH, Lee HK, Moon JG. Chronic subdural hematomas: a comparative study of three types of operative procedures. *J Korean Neurosurg Soc* 2009; **46**: 210–214.

Lega BC, Danish SF, Malhotra NR, Sonnad SS, Stein SC. Choosing the best operation for chronic subdural hematoma: a decision analysis. *J Neurosurg* 2009 October 30.

Lind CR, Lind CJ, Mee EW. Reduction in the number of repeated operations for the treatment of subacute and chronic subdural hematomas by placement of subdural drains. *Journal of Neurosurgery* 2003; **99**: 44–46.

Markwalder TM. Chronic subdural hematomas: a review. *J Neurosurg* 1981; **54**: 637–645.

Markwalder TM, Seiler RW. Chronic subdural hematomas: to drain or not to drain? *Neurosurgery* 1985; **16**: 185–188.

Mondorf Y, Abu-Owaimer M, Gaab MR, Oertel JM. Chronic subdural hematoma—Craniotomy versus burr hole trepanation. *Br J Neurosurg* 2009; **23**: 612–616.

Mori K, Maeda M. Surgical treatment of chronic subdural hematoma in 500 consecutive cases: clinical characteristics, surgical outcome, complications, and recurrence rate. *Neurologia Medico-Chirurgica* 2001; **41**: 371–381.

Santarius T, Lawton R, Kirkpatrick PJ, Hutchinson PJ. The management of primary chronic subdural haematoma: a questionnaire survey of practice in the United Kingdom and the Republic of Ireland. *Br J Neurosurg* 2008; **22**: 529–534.

Svien HJ, Gelety JE. On the surgical management of encapsulated chronic subdural hematoma. A comparison of the results of membranectomy and simple evacuation. *Journal of Neurosurgery* 1964; **21**: 172–177.

Tsutsumi K, Maeda K, Iijima A, Usui M, Okada Y, Kirino T. The relationship of preoperative magnetic resonance imaging findings and closed system drainage in the recurrence of chronic subdural hematoma. *J Neurosurgery* 1997; **87**: 870–875.

Wakai S, Hashimoto K, Watanabe N, Inoh S, Ochiai C, Nagai M. Efficacy of closed-system drainage in treating chronic subdural hematoma: a prospective comparative study. *Neurosurgery* 1990; **26**: 771–773.

Weigel R, Schmiedek P, Krauss JK. Outcome of contemporary surgery for chronic subdural haematoma: evidence based review. *J Neurol Neurosurg Psychiatry* 2003; **74**: 937–943.

3.4 Intracranial pressure monitoring in head injury

Details of studies

Intracranial pressure monitoring was introduced into neurosurgical practice in the second half of the 20th century (Guillaume and Hanny, 1951; Lundberg, 1960). However, two studies carried out in the 1970s and early 1980s at the Medical College of Virginia in Richmond, Virginia, USA, firmly established the role of ICP monitoring in head-injured patients (Miller et al., 1977; Miller et al., 1981).

Study references

Main studies

Miller JD, Becker DP, Ward JD, Sullivan HG, Adams WE, Rosner MJ. Significance of intracranial hypertension in severe head injury. *J Neurosurg* 1977; **47**: 503–516.

Miller JD, Butterworth JF, Gudeman SK, Faulkner JE, Choi SC, Selhorst JB, Harbison JW, Lutz HA, Young HF, Becker DP. Further experience in the management of severe head injury. *J Neurosurg* 1981; **54**: 289–299.

Related references

Guillaume J, Hanny P. Manometrie intacranienne continue: Interet de la methode et premiers resultats. *Rev Neurol* 1951; **84**: 131–142.

Lundberg N. Continuous recording and control of in neurosurgical practice. *Acta Psychiatr Neurol Scand* 1960; **3**: 190–193.

Narayan RK, Kishore PRS, Becker DP, Ward JD, Enas GG, Greenberg RP, Da Silva AD, Lipper MH, Choi SC, Mayhall CG, Lutz HA, Young HF. Intracranial pressure: to monitor or not to monitor? A review of our experience with severe head injury. *J Neurosurg* 1982; **56**: 650–659.

Study designs

- Miller *et al.* (1977) and Narayan *et al.* (1982) were retrospective case series analyses.
- Miller *et al.* (1981) was a prospective consecutive series analysis.

	Miller *et al.* (1977)	Miller *et al.* (1981)
Class of evidence	III	III
Number of patients	160	225
Follow-up	Retrospective analysis	1 year
Outcomes	Death and disability	Death and disability
Eligibility	Blunt head injury Motor score <6 on GCS No evidence of brain death	Severe head injury V2, M3 or less on the GCS No evidence of brain death Gunshot wounds and patients without spontaneous respiration were excluded
Number of centres	1	1

- ICP recordings were made by transducing from a ventricular catheter placed in the frontal horn of one of the lateral ventricles.

- In the first study, the initial threshold for treating raised ICP was a sustained rise over 40 mmHg. However, by the end of the study this was reduced to 30 mmHg and in the later studies the threshold was set at an ICP of 25 mmHg for over 15 min.
- Outcomes were assessed using the 5 point GOS with a good outcome being defined as moderate disability or good recovery and a poor outcome being defined as a significant disability, vegetative state, or death.

Results

Miller *et al.* (1977)

- ICP >40 mmHg on admission was associated with a poor outcome: 69% mortality and only 25% good outcome ($p < 0.01$).
- Low ICP on admission (<10 mmHg) was associated with much better outcomes: 14% mortality and 78% survived to a good outcome ($p < 0.05$).
- These findings of early ICP recording were even more significant when applied to patients with diffuse brain injury. In patients with mass lesions, only very high ICP (>40 mmHg) was associated with a poor outcome.
- Patients with diffuse injuries who experienced delayed elevations in ICP >20 mmHg had a greater proportion of poor outcomes (46%) compared to those whose ICP remained below <20 mmHg (21%, $p < 0.02$).
- 50% of fatalities were associated with uncontrolled intracranial hypertension.

Miller *et al.* (1981)

- The authors reported a significant correlation between ICP control and outcome ($p < 0.001$: more patients with a well-controlled ICP (<20 mmHg) throughout had a much better outcome (74% good outcome, 18% mortality) compared to patients with raised but reducible ICPs (55% good outcome, 26% mortality) and those with uncontrolled ICP rises (only 3% good outcome, and 92% mortality).

Conclusions

Miller *et al.* (1977)

- Elevated ICP is related to poor outcome in severely head-injured patients.

Miller *et al.* (1981)

- Even moderate intracranial hypertension is associated with a poor outcome in patients with severe head injuries.

Critique

Lundberg *et al.* reported a preliminary assessment of continuous ICP monitoring in a series of 30 patients in 1965 (Lundberg *et al.*, 1965). In addition, Johnston and Jennett emphasized that ICP monitoring in head-injured patients might be used to aid diagnosis, guide management, and predict outcomes (Johnston and Jennett, 1973). However, until the studies from Virginia there was a poor correlation between ICP and outcome in severely head-injured patients as reported in the literature. These two studies are landmark studies because they led to the widespread use of ICP monitoring in head-injured patients. However, the value of managing patients with ICP monitoring has been challenged, particularly as there appeared to be similar outcomes in patients managed without (Stuart *et al.*, 1983). The absence of a randomized trial is often cited to suggest that there is no evidence for the value of ICP monitoring and that its use may inappropriately prolong ventilation and intensive therapy in severely injured patients (Cremer *et al.*, 2005). In a survey of 67 centres from 12 European countries, patients who were ICP monitored appeared to have more interventions and poorer outcomes than those who were not (Stocchetti *et al.*, 2001). In a review of the available evidence, Stocchetti *et al.* have outlined three potential conclusions regarding ICP monitoring (Stocchetti *et al.*, 2001). The pessimistic view that it is not of proven value and the decision to monitor is a matter of personal opinion; the nihilistic view that it is an invasive procedure without proven benefit and should not be used; and the optimistic view that benefits may be demonstrated in large trials. Although there is a body of support for a large clinical trial, the widespread use of ICP monitoring means that it is likely to form an integral part of the intensive management of severely head-injured patients (Chieregato, 2007). If such trials are ever carried out it may be that refractory ICP and response to treatment of raised ICP may prove to be better predictors of neurological outcome than absolute ICP values (Treggiari *et al.*, 2007).

Chieregato A. Randomized clinical trial of intracranial pressure monitoring after severe head injury. *Crit Care Med* 2007; **35**: 673–674.

Cremer OL, van Dijk GW, van Wensen E, Brekelmans GJ, Moons KG, Leenen LP, Kalkman CJ. Effect of intracranial pressure monitoring and targeted intensive care on functional outcome after severe head injury. *Crit Care Med* 2005; **33**: 2207–2213.

Johnston IH, Jennett B. The place of intracranial pressure monitoring in neurosurgical practice. *Acta Neurochir* 1973; **29**: 53–63.

Lundberg NL, Troupp H, Lorin H. Continuous recording of the ventricular-fluid pressure in patients with severe acute traumatic brain injury. A preliminary report. *J Neurosurg* 1965; **22**: 581–590.

Stocchetti N, Penny KI, Dearden M, Braakman R, Cohadon F, Iannotti F, Lapierre F, Karimi A, Maas A Jr, Murray GD, Ohman J, Persson L, Servadei F, Teasdale GM, Trojanowski T, Unterberg A; European Brain Injury Consortium. Intensive care management of head-injured patients in Europe: a survey from the European brain injury consortium. *Intensive Care Med* 2001; **27**: 400–406.

Stocchetti N, Lonhgi L, Zanier ER. Intracranial pressure monitoring for traumatic brain injury: available evidence and clinical implications. *Minerva Anestesiol* 2008; **74**: 197–203.

Stuart GG, Merry GS, Smith JA, Yelland JD. Severe head injury managed without intracranial pressure monitoring. *J Neurosurg* 1983 Oct; **59**(4): 601–605.

Treggiari MM, Schutz N, Yanez ND, Romand JA. Role of intracranial pressure values and patterns in predicting outcome in traumatic brain injury: a systematic review. *Neurocrit Care* 2007; **6**: 104–112.

3.5 **Steroids in head injury**

Details of study

The Corticosteroids Randomization After Significant Head Injury (CRASH) trial is the largest multi-centre, international randomized controlled trial looking at the effect of methyl prednisolone on the risk of death and disability after head injury.

Study references

Main study

CRASH trial collaborators. Final results of MRC CRASH, a randomised placebo-controlled trial of intravenous corticosteroid in adults with head injury - outcomes at 6 months. *Lancet* 2005; **365**: 1957–1959.

CRASH trial collaborators. Lancet. Effects of intravenous corticosteroids on death within 14 days in 10008 adults with clinically significant head injury (MRC CRASH trial). *Lancet* 2004; **364**: 1321–1328.

Related references

Alderson P, Roberts I. Corticosteroids for acute traumatic brain injury. *Cochrane Database of Syst Rev* 2005; Issue 1. Art. No: CD000196.

Bracken MB. CRASH (Corticosteroids Randomisation after Significant Head Injury): Landmark and storm warning. *Neurosurgery* 2005; **57**: 1300–1302.

Peto R. Possible explanations of the CRASH result. *Lancet* 2005; **364**: 213.

Study design

- Placebo-controlled randomized trial (PRCT)

Class of evidence	I
Randomization	Methyl prednisolone infusion versus placebo
Number of patients	10,008
Follow-up	Primary outcomes: 1. Death within 2 weeks of injury 2. Death and disability at 6 months
	Secondary outcomes: None
	Percentage of patients followed up at each stage? 1. 100 % at 2 weeks 2. 96.7% at 6 months
Number of centres	239 centres in 49 countries worldwide
Stratification	Presence or absence of generalized motor seizures

- CRASH set out to recruit 20,000 patients but was stopped after 10,008 were randomized.
- There were more patients in CRASH than all previous trials looking at methyl prednisolone in head injury combined.

- Methyl prednisolone was administered within 8 h of injury with a loading dose of 2 g (in 100 mL) over 1 h, followed by a 48-h maintenance dose.

Outcome measures

Primary endpoints

- Death within 2 weeks
- Death or disability (assessed with a questionnaire version of GOS) at 6 months

Results

Outcome		Methyl prednisolone group	Placebo group	Statistical significance
Death within 2 weeks		21.1%	17.9%	$p = 0.001$
Death at 6 months		25.7%	22.3%	$p = 0.0001$
Disability at 6 months	Severe	11.9%	13.6%	None
	Moderate	17.6%	16.9%	None

Conclusions

Steroids should not be routinely used in the treatment of head injury.

Critique

The CRASH trial is the first large-scale randomized controlled trial in severe head-injured patients. Although many other previous trials had been carried out (over 15), meta-analysis of previous trials had shown that there might be a potential benefit in the use steroids to treat head injury. However, once the CRASH trial is included in this meta-analysis the data support the conclusions of the CRASH trial. The CRASH trial conclusion could perhaps be more specific in that the results do not support the routine use of methyl prednisolone in the treatment of head injury rather than all steroids *per se*.

The CRASH trial was criticized for testing only a small effect thus requiring such large numbers to be recruited. The trial was planned to detect a 2% reduction in mortality from 15% to 13% and was planned for the randomization of 20,000 patients. The CRASH trial is the largest trial in head injury to date and included more patients than all other trials combined that had previously addressed the role of steroids in head injury. In addition, CRASH is the largest trial of severe head injury as it included 3944 such patients. CRASH has conclusively answered the question regarding methyl prednisolone in the treatment of head injury. Furthermore, the massive population of head-injured patients included in the CRASH trial has allowed for the development of prognostic models for predicting outcome. The MRC CRASH Trial Collaborators developed two web-based prognostic models that can be applied to individual patients in order to predict outcome (MRC CRASH Trial Collaborators, 2008). This allows for the application of models based on population-based data to individual practice. In addition, this may be useful for prognostic stratification in future trials.

The CRASH trial has allowed investigators to move on to research in other therapeutic modalities for head injury. A CRASH2 trial is now underway looking into the effects of tranexamic acid on survival following head injury. The ProTECT study is now underway to look at the effects of progesterone in head injury. The Phase II results of ProTECT have been published and no significant adverse effects were seen with progesterone (Wright *et al.*, 2007). The ProTECT study has laid the foundations for a much larger multi-centre study into the effect of progesterone in the treatment of head injury. There has also been a trial investigating the neuroprotective effects of magnesium sulphate infusions after traumatic brain injury.

Alderson P, Roberts I. Corticosteroids for acute traumatic brain injury. *Cochrane Database of Syst Rev* 2005; Issue 1. Art. No: CD000196.

Bracken MB. CRASH (Corticosteroids Randomisation after Significant Head Injury): Landmark and storm warning. *Neurosurgery* 2005; 57: 1300–1302.

Peto R. Possible explanations of the CRASH result. *Lancet* 2005; 364: 213.

Wright DW, Kellermann AL, Hertzberg VS, Clark PL, Frankel M, Goldstein FC, Salomone JP, Dent LL, Harris OA, Ander DS, Lowery DW, Patel MM, Denson DD, Gordon AB, Wald MM, Gupta S, Hoffman SW, Stein DG. ProTECT: A randomised clinical trial of progesterone for acute traumatic brain injury. *Annals Emerg Med* 2007; 49: 391–402.

3.6 **Barbiturates in head injury**

Details of study

The study by Eisenberg *et al.* is the first randomized controlled trial to assess the efficacy of pentobarbital to treat elevated ICP in severely head-injured patients. Although two previous trials had been carried out to assess pentobarbital to prevent rises in ICP in these patients, neither had revealed a benefit (Schwartz *et al.*, 1984; Ward *et al.*, 1985). The trial by Eisenberg *et al.* was carried out over a 5-year period between 1982 and 1987 in the United States.

Study references

Main study

Eisenberg HM, Frankowski RF, Contant CF, Marshall LF, Walker MD. High-dose barbiturates control elevated intracranial pressure in patients with severe head injury. *J Neurosurg* 1988; **69**: 15–23.

Related references

Roberts I. Barbiturates for acute traumatic brain injury. *Cochrane Database Syst Rev* 2000; **2**: CD000033.

Schwartz ML, Tator CH, Rowed DW, Reif SR, Meguro K, Andrews DF. The University of Toronto Head Injury Treatment Study: a prospective, randomised comparison of pentobarbital and mannitol. *Can J Neurol Sci* 1984; **11**: 434–440.

Ward JD, Becker DP, Miller JD, Choi SC, Marmarou A, Wood C, Newlon PG, Keenan R. Failure of prophylactic barbiturate coma in the treatment of severe head injury. *J Neurosurg* 1985; **62**: 383–388.

Study design

- ◆ PRCT

Class of evidence	I
Randomization	Best conventional therapy versus pentobarbital
Number of patients	73
Follow-up	6 months
	Primary endpoints: Response to treatment
	Other endpoints: Survival; GOS
Number of centres	5
Stratification	Medical complications Time to randomization Initial GCS

- ◆ Inclusion criteria: GCS 4–7 post-resuscitation; age 15–50 years; serum osmolality/ ≥315 mOsm/kg; mannitol given within 1 h prior to randomization.

- ◆ Exclusion criteria: GCS 3; fixed pupils; pregnancy.

- ◆ Conventional therapy standardized across all five centres.

- ◆ Intracranial mass lesions, haematomas, and accessible contusions resected.

- Patients with uncontrolled ICP despite best conventional therapy (BCT) received pentobarbital (titrated to serum concentration) plus continued BCT.
- ICP randomization criteria based on ICP levels and length of time ICP raised, e.g. randomization for closed head injury if ICP >25 mmHg (30 min), >30 mmHg (15 min), or 40 mmHg (1 min). Lower values used for open injuries.
- Response to treatment in patients with closed head injury defined as successful if ICP <20 mmHg for 48 h (lower value for open head injury).
- Failed reductions in ICP or severe clinical deterioration (e.g. fixed pupil, or death) were defined as unsuccessful treatment.
- Patients whose ICP remained uncontrolled in the BCT arm were allowed to cross-over to pentobarbital treatment.

Results

	BCT	BCT + pentobarbital	Benefit ratio of pentobarbital + BCT:BCT
Control of ICP in all patients (% of patients)	16.7%	32.4%	2:1
Control of ICP in patients with cardiovascular complications prior to randomization (% of patients)	9%	40%	4:1

- Multiple logistic model statistical analysis revealed a significant positive treatment effect of pentobarbital ($p = 0.04$).
- Significant effects of timing of randomization were also found: twice as many.
- Uncontrolled ICP was robustly associated with death in both treatment arms (>90% of patients with controlled ICP survived).

Conclusions

High-dose barbiturates are an appropriate adjunct in the control of raised ICP in severely head-injured patients.

Critique

Severe head injury is associated with extremely high morbidity and mortality. Although the primary insult is not treatable, prevention of secondary injury due to the resultant cascade of insults may be feasible. The trial by Eisenberg *et al.* aimed to evaluate the role of barbiturate therapy in this regard. Unfortunately, only 12% of patients considered for randomization met the entry criteria and the total number of patients in the trial is still quite low. Nonetheless, the trial was still a multi-centre trial with standardized treatment regimes. Survival was not the primary outcome measure, but rather control of ICP. This was primarily to avoid the ethical dilemma of not using barbiturates when ICP reached potentially lethal levels. The authors pointed out that there is a possibility that raised ICP and outcome are both predetermined by the pathology of severe head injury. However, ICP >20 mmHg had been consistently found to be significantly associated with poor outcome in previous studies of severely head-injured patients, which provided an acceptable rationale to design a trial with ICP as primary outcome.

As stated above, two previous studies on prophylactic efficacy of barbiturates to control ICP had been performed that did not suggest a benefit (Schwartz et al., 1984; Ward et al., 1985). The trial by Eisenberg et al., therefore, has provided the first evidence that barbiturates may be effective in controlling ICP in severely head-injured patients. However, the debate regarding the relationship between ICP and outcome is still ongoing. In a Cochrane review of all published trials involving barbiturates, Roberts concluded that although barbiturates controlled ICP in severely head-injured patients, there was no evidence to support any beneficial effect on outcome (Roberts, 2000).

Roberts I. Barbiturates for acute traumatic brain injury. *Cochrane Database Syst Rev* 2000; **2**: CD000033.

Schwartz ML, Tator CH, Rowed DW, Reif SR, Meguro K, Andrews DF. The University of Toronto Head Injury Treatment Study: a prospective, randomised comparison of pentobarbital and mannitol. *Can J Neurol Sci* 1984; **11**: 434–440.

Ward JD, Becker DP, Miller JD, Choi SC, Marmarou A, Wood C, Newlon PG, Keenan R. Failure of prophylactic barbiturate coma in the treatment of severe head injury. *J Neurosurg* 1985; **62**: 383–388.

3.7 **Hyperosmolar therapy for control of raised intracranial pressure in head injury**

Details of studies

Mannitol and saline are the two most widely used hyperosmolar therapies available to control raised intracranial pressure in head injury. The efficacy of mannitol has been studied by a series of reasonably sized randomized controlled clinical trials. The first of these was carried out in Toronto, Canada, and compared mannitol with pentobarbital (Schwartz *et al.*, 1984). The second compared mannitol to saline, as opposed to hypertonic saline (Sayre *et al.*, 1996). The third trial, carried out in North Carolina, USA, included two regimens both of which used mannitol but compared two different sets of parameters (physiological measurements versus ICP) to guide administration (Smith *et al.*, 1986). A further three trials have been carried out by Cruz *et al.* in San Paolo, Brazil (Cruz *et al.*, 2001; Cruz *et al.*, 2002; Cruz *et al.*, 2004). These three trials assessed the effects of early high-dose mannitol in three different groups of severely head-injured patients: patients with surgically treated acute subdural haematomas (Cruz *et al.*, 2001); patients with acute temporal intraparenchymal haemorrhages (Cruz *et al.*, 2002); and patients with severe diffuse brain injury (Cruz *et al.*, 2004). These trials show a large variation in their design and in the primary question they set out to evaluate. Notwithstanding this we have included them all here as they are all randomized studies using mannitol in head-injured patients. The efficacy of hypertonic saline has also been evaluated in comparison with Ringer's lactate in a large trial carried out in Melbourne, Australia (Cooper *et al.*, 2004). In addition, one small study from Marseille, France, has compared hypertonic saline with mannitol (Vialet *et al.*, 2003).

Study references

Main studies

Mannitol

Cruz J, Minoja G, Okuchi K. Improving clinical outcomes from acute subdural hematomas with the emergency preoperative administration of high doses of mannitol: a randomized trial. *Neurosurgery* 2001; **49**: 864–871.

Cruz J, Minoja G, Okuchi K. Major clinical and physiological benefits of early high doses of mannitol for intraparenchymal temporal lobe hemorrhages with abnormal pupillary widening: a randomised trial. *Neurosurgery* 2002; **51**: 628–637.

Cruz J, Minoja G, Okuchi K, Facco E. Successful use of the new high-dose mannitol treatment in patients with Glasgow Coma Scale scores of 3 and bilateral abnormal pupillary widening: a randomized trial. *Neurosurgery* 2004; **100**: 376–383.

Sayre MR, Daily SW, Stern SA, Storer DL, van Loveren HR, Hurst JM. Out-of-hospital administration of mannitol does not change systolic blood pressure. *Acad Emerg Med* 1996; **3**: 840–848.

Schwartz M, Tator C, Rowed DW, Reid SR, Meguro K, Andrews DF. The University of Toronto Head Injury Treatment Study: a prospective randomised comparison of pento-barbital and mannitol. *Can J Neurol Sci* 1984; **11**: 434–440.

Smith HP, Kelly DL Jr, McWhorter JM, Armstrong D, Johnson RD, Transou C, Howard G. Comparison of mannitol regimens in patients with severe head injury undergoing intracranial pressure monitoring. *J Neurosurg* 1986; **65**: 820–824.

Hypertonic saline and mannitol versus hypertonic saline

Cooper DJ, Myles PS, McDermott FT, Murray LJ, Laidlaw J, Cooper G, Tremayne AB, Bernard SS, Ponsford J for the HTS Study Investigators. Prehospital hypertonic saline resuscitation of patients with hypotension and severe traumatic brain injury: a randomized controlled trial. *JAMA* 2004 17; **291**: 1350–1357.

Vialet R, Albanese J, Thomachot L, Antonini R, Bourgouin A, Alliez B, Martin C. Isovolume hypertonic solutes (sodium chloride or mannitol) in the treatment of refractory posttraumatic intracranial hypertension: 2 mgL/kg 7.5% saline is more effective than 2 ml/kg 20% mannitol. *Critical Care Medicine* 2003; **31**: 1683–1687.

Related reference

Wakai A, Roberts I, Schierhout G. Mannitol for acute traumatic brain injury. *Cochrane Database Syst Rev* 2007; **24**: CD001049.

Study designs

- All PRCTs but blinding varied between trials.

	Hyperosmolar Treatment Regime
Schwartz et al. (1984)	1 g/kg of 20% mannitol given initially (followed by incremental titration to achieve ICP control) and pentobarbital as an IV bolus of up to 10 mL/kg followed by a continuous infusion at 0.5–3 mg/kg/h
Smith et al. (1986)	Mannitol administration guided according to neurological signs and physiological parameters or gave a 250 mL bolus of 20% mannitol for ICP >25 mmHg followed by incremental boluses as required
Sayre et al. (1996)	Pre-hospital administration of 5 ml/kg of 20% mannitol compared with administration of 5 mL/kg of 0.9% saline
Cruz et al. (2001, 2002, 2004)	Early high-dose mannitol (HDM) at 1.4 g/kg compared with conventional-dose mannitol (CDM) at 0.7 g/kg
Cooper et al. (2004)	A 250 mL infusion of 7.5% hypertonic saline was compared with 250 mL of Ringer's lactate (both through a peripheral line)
Vialet et al. (2003)	2 mL/kg body weight of 20% mannitol compared with 2 mL/kg body weight of 7.5% hypertonic saline solution (HSS) given when either ICP >25 mmHg, or CPP <70 mmHg for more than 5 min

- The trial by Schwartz *et al.* contained two cohorts of patients: those without intracranial haematomas and those with elevated ICP following haematoma evacuation.
- The three trials by Cruz *et al.* looked at three different cohorts of patients respectively: those with subdural haematomas (ASDH); those with temporal intraparenchymal haematomas (temporal IPH); and those with diffuse brain injury (DBI).
- Vialet *et al.* defined treatment failure as an inability to reduce ICP below 25 mmHg or to increase cerebral perfusion pressure (CPP) to >70 mmHg after two sequential boluses of hyperosmolar fluid.

Results

Schwartz et al. (1984)

	Mannitol	Pentobarbital	Statistical significance
Mortality in patients with ICP elevation but no haematoma	41%	77%	$p < 0.05$
Mortality in patients with raised ICP after haematoma evacuation	43%	40%	None

Smith et al. (1986)

	ICP-guided mannitol therapy	Empirical mannitol therapy	Statistical significance
Mortality	35%	42.5%	None

- Mean ICP was 5.5 mmHg lower in the empirically treated group compared to the ICP-guided group ($p < 0.05$).

Sayre et al. (1996)

- After 2 h, those patients receiving mannitol had a lower systolic blood pressure compared to placebo (116 ± 24 mmHg versus 142 ± 25 mmHg, $p < 0.003$).
- However, there was no overall difference in blood pressure between mannitol and placebo groups over the whole 2-h observation period.

Cruz et al. (2001, 2002, 2004)

- 6-month clinical outcomes.

	Cruz et al. (2001) (ASDH)			Cruz et al. (2002) (Temporal IPH)			Cruz et al. (2004) (DBI)		
	HDM	CDM	Statistical significance	HDM	CDM	Statistical significance	HDM	CDM	Statistical significance
Good recovery or moderate disability	69.2%	46.0%		61.1%	33.3%		43.5%	9.5%	
Severe disability	13.2%	24.1%	$p < 0.01$	15.3%	24.6%	$p < 0.005$	56.5%	90.5%	$p < 0.02$
Vegetative state or death	17.6%	29.9%		23.6%	42%				
Mortality	14.3%	25.3%		39.1%	66.7%		19.4%	36.2%	

- In their 2001 study of patients with ASDH, Cruz *et al.* reported a significant improvement in abnormal pre-operative pupillary widening in the HDM group ($p < 0.0001$).
- In their 2002 study of patients with traumatic temporal IPH, Cruz *et al.* reported that HDM resulted in significant improvements in pre-operative abnormal pupillary widening both bilaterally ($p < 0.03$) and unilaterally ($p < 0.01$).
- In their 2004 study of patients with DBI, Cruz *et al.* reported a significant early improvement of bilateral abnormal pupillary widening in the HDM group ($p < 0.02$).

Cooper *et al.* (2004)

	Hypertonic saline	Ringer's lactate	Statistical significance
Good recovery or moderate disability	37.7%	19.3%	None
Severe disability	9.6%	30.4%	None
Survival to discharge	55%	47%	None

- 6-month clinical outcomes.

Vialet *et al.* (2003)

	Hypertonic saline	Mannitol	Statistical significance
Number of episodes ICP >25 mmHg	6.8	13.3	$p < 0.02$
Total duration of episodes	62 min	95 min	$p < 0.04$
Treatment failure	10%	70%	$p < 0.01$

- Mean daily outcomes.
- There was no significant difference in mortality or GOS between the two treatment arms.

Conclusions

Schwartz *et al.* (1984)

- There is no difference between mannitol and pentobarbital in the treatment of intracranial hypertension following head injury.
- Pentobarbital may be harmful in head-injured patients without intracranial haematomas.

Smith *et al.* (1986)

- Regular, frequent administration of mannitol may result in better overall control of ICP than waiting until ICP rises above 25 mmHg.

Sayre *et al.* (1996)

- Out-of-hospital administration of 1.0 g/kg of mannitol to multiple-trauma head-injured patients is not associated with significant hypotension.

Cruz *et al.* (2001, 2002, 2004)

♦ Early administration of HDM leads to significant improvements and better clinical outcomes in patients with ASDH, traumatic temporal IPH, and DBI.

Cooper *et al.* (2004)

♦ Hypertonic saline in the pre-hospital setting for severely head-injured patients is no better than conventional fluids alone for resuscitating hypotensive patients or improving neurological outcomes at 6 months.

Vialet *et al.* (2003)

♦ Hypertonic saline was more effective in controlling refractory intracranial hypertension than mannitol in patients with severe head injury.

Critique

The utility of mannitol in controlling intracranial pressure has been well established. Its effect on outcome has been more variable. Early data on hypertonic saline are similar to that for mannitol.

The study by Schwartz *et al.* focused predominantly on the effect of mannitol on ICP control. This study has been criticized because it allowed cross-over between groups if there was subsequent raised ICP. Nonetheless, the finding that pentobarbital may have been harmful in the patients in this study has contributed considerably to the widespread use of mannitol to control ICP in head-injured patients. The trial by Smith *et al.* assessed whether there was any benefit in the use of ICP monitoring to guide the use of mannitol in severely head-injured patients. They found that there was no statistically significant difference in either mortality or neurological outcome using ICP monitoring. However, the authors did suggest that their finding that mean ICP was lower in the empirically treated group might indicate that better ICP control could be achieved with small regular doses of mannitol rather than waiting until ICP rises above 25 mmHg.

In the study by Sayre *et al.*, death was not the primary outcome as they powered their study to detect a drop in systolic BP to <90 mmHg (83% power). The study was not, therefore, powered to detect a difference in survival at 2 h. However, as hypotension is associated with a doubling in mortality in patients with severe head injury their chosen endpoint is a reasonable one (Gentleman and Jennett, 1981). Cooper *et al.*'s study was powered to detect a single grade change in GOS, which represents a meaningful clinical difference in outcome. This trial is also, therefore, a landmark trial for being the first resuscitation fluid trial to measure neurological outcome as a primary outcome. One of the weaknesses of Cooper *et al.*'s study is that it included multiple-injured patients, which raised concerns regarding whether conclusions could be extrapolated to patients, which isolated head injuries. Although this is a concern, Cooper *et al.* reported that the outcomes of patients were better than would have been predicted from trauma severity scores.

The trials by Sayre *et al.* and Cooper *et al.* are particularly noteworthy in that they are examples of randomized blinded trials conducted for interventions in the pre-hospital setting.

Lewis has emphasized that trials conducted for therapies in this setting are particularly difficult because of difficulties with availability of personnel, equipment, space, and lighting (Lewis, 2004). Lewis also highlights that such trials face ethical issues regarding consent because of the need to show that patients are in a life-threatening situation and that available treatment options are unproven or are believed to be ineffective. Only in these circumstances can prospective written informed consent be bypassed to enrol patients into a trial.

The patients in the first HDM trial by Cruz et al. had acute traumatic subdural haematomas requiring emergency evacuation. In such circumstances, common practice in most centres is to give mannitol to patients with pupillary abnormalities, and nothing to patients with normal pupillary responses, yet all these patients initially received low-dose (0.6–0.7 g/kg) mannitol regardless. A recent Cochrane review questioned the integrity of Cruz's data, in particular its randomization (Wakai et al., 2007). Wilberger found it particularly noteworthy that the mortality rate reported for this study is the lowest ever observed (Wilberger, 2001). Marion indicated that the management by Cruz pays close attention to the standardization of care and the close monitoring of physiological parameters and control of cerebral perfusion and oxygenation (Marion, 2001). However, Marion also raised concerns that statistical analysis did not take into account confounding variables such as the initial GCS. Concerns have been raised regarding the unusual lack of hypotensive episodes in patients included in the trials reported by Cruz (Valadka, 2002). Perhaps the most intriguing question resulting from Cruz's work, however, is how a single early HDM bolus might lead to such long-term beneficial effects. Notwithstanding this, Zygun has criticized the lack of any blinding that would have been feasible seeing as the HDM was a single one-off bolus given early in the management of the patient (Zygun, 2004). More serious concerns regarding the integrity of Cruz's work have been expressed in the literature (Roberts et al., 2007). However, these studies have not been formally retracted from the literature and so they have been included here. We leave it to the reader to determine for themselves whether the data should be considered reliable.

Cooper's study comparing mannitol with hypertonic saline has been criticized for being powered to detect a 20% improvement in GOSE. At the lower end of the GOSE, this could represent a change from death to persistent vegetative state (Zygun, 2004a; Zygun, 2004b). Zygun has expressed the view that the attainment of a functional neurologic status would be deemed a more meaningful outcome by most clinicians. It is possible that a higher than normal serum sodium on arrival in hospital in the hypertonic saline group could have affected blinding in this study.

Vialet's trial had small numbers of patients, but was sufficiently powered as repeated measures were taken from each patient. However, Vialet's small numbers raise concerns about case heterogeneity, and the extremely poor outcomes at 90 days (all patients in the study were dead or severely disabled). This raises questions about whether the study group was appropriately representative or managed optimally otherwise.

The evidence for hyperosmolar therapy is limited both in number of studies undertaken and in delineating several aspects of its use. There remains little evidence about whether hyperosmolar therapies should be given as boluses or continuous infusions, whether there is an optimal dose, an optimal rate, whether losses from diuresis should be replaced, whether clinical thresholds should be guided by intracranial pressure or according to fixed schedules (and if so when they should be best timed), and whether serum osmolarity alterations alter outcomes.

All these studies are landmark studies as they have greatly contributed to our knowledge regarding the use of hypertonic osmotic therapies in head-injured patients. Nonetheless, the mechanism of action of these agents remains to be fully elucidated. Although osmotic tissue dehydration may still play some role in the action of hyperosmolar therapies, they work primarily through immediate rheological effects, diluting the blood and increasing the deformability of erythrocytes, thereby decreasing blood viscosity and promoting cerebral blood flow. Thus, mechanistic studies suggest that bolus administration and replacing urinary losses are best practice.

There is limited clinical evidence that successive mannitol boluses accumulate in cerebral tissue and exacerbate intracranial pressure and that cumulative hyperosmolar effects can have detrimental neurological sequelae (Wakai et al., 2007). Theoretical concerns with hypertonic saline include the development of central pontine myelinolysis and rapid brain shrinkage leading to tearing of bridging vessels. However, pontine myelinolysis is seen if chronic hyponatraemia is rapidly corrected, and hyponatraemia is usually not an immediate problem in acute severe head injury. There is no evidence that hypertonic saline is superior to mannitol and both are in widespread clinical use.

Gentleman D, Jennett B. Hazards of inter-hospital transfer of comatose head-injured patients. *Lancet* 1981; 2: 853–854.

Lewis RJ. Prehospital care of the multiply injured patient. The challenge of figuring out what works. *JAMA* 2004; **291**: 1382–1383.

Marion DW. Improved outcomes with high dose mannitol treatment: comments. *Neurosurgery* 2001; **49**: 871.

Roberts I, Smith R, Evans S. Doubts over head injury studies. *BMJ* 2007; **334**: 392–394.

Wakai A, Roberts I, Schierhout G. Mannitol for acute traumatic brain injury. *Cochrane Database Syst Rev* 2007; **24**: CD001049.

Valadka AB. Emergency benefits of high-dose mannitol: comments. *Neurosurgery* 2002; **51**: 637–638.

Wilberger JE. Improved outcomes with high dose mannitol treatment: comments. *Neurosurgery* 2001; **49**: 871.

Zygun D. High-dose mannitol. *J Neurosurg* 2004a; **101**: 567.

Zygun D. Hypertonic saline for prehospital treatment of traumatic brain injury. *JAMA* 2004b; **24**: 2943.

3.8 **Hypothermia in head injury**
Details of study

The multi-centre randomized trial by Clifton *et al.* (2001) of treatment with hypothermia for patients with severe traumatic brain injury (TBI) patients aimed to determine the efficacy of therapeutic hypothermia within 8 h of injury. The trial was carried out in the United States between 1994 and 1998.

Study reference

Main study

Clifton GL, Miller ER, Choi SC, Levin HS, McCauley S, Smith K, Muizelaar JP, Wagner FC, Marion DW, Luerssen TG, Chestnut RM, Schwartz M. Lack of effect of induction of hypothermia after acute brain injury. *N Engl J Med* 2001; **344**: 556–563.

Related references

Harris OA, Colford JM, Good MC, Matx PG. The role of hypothermia in the management of severe brain injury. A meta-analysis. *Arch Neurol* 2002; **59**: 1077–1083.

Henderson WR, Dhingra VK, Chittock DR, Fenwick JC, Ronco JJ. Hypothermia in the management of traumatic brain injury. A systematic review and meta-analysis. *Intensive Care Med* 2003; **29**: 1637–1644.

Hutchison JS, Ward RE, Lacroix JL, Hebert PC, Barnes MA, Bohn DJ, Dirks PB, Douchette S, Fergusson D. Gottesman R, Joffe AR, Kirkpalani HM, Meyer PG, Morris KP, Moher D, Singh RN, Skippen PW for the Hypothermia Pediatric Head Injury Trial Investigators and the Canadian Critical Care Trials Group. Hypothermia therapy after traumatic brain injury in children. *N Engl J Med* 2008; **358**: 2447–2456.

McIntyre LA, Fergusson DA, Hérbert PC, Moher D, Hutchison JS. Prolonged therapeutic hypothermia after traumatic brain injury in adults. *JAMA* 2003; **289**: 2992–2999.

Shiozaki T, Hayakata T, Taneda T Nakajima Y, Hashiguchi N, Fujimi S, Nakamori Y, Tanaka H, Shimazu T, Sugimoto H. A multicenter prospective randomised controlled trial of the efficacy of mild hypothermia for severely head injured patients with low intracranial pressure. *J Neurosurg* 2001; **94**: 50–54.

Study design

◆ Multi-centre randomized controlled trial (RT)

Class of evidence	II
Randomization	Hypothermia versus normothermia
Number of patients	392 patients
Follow-up	6 months
	Primary outcome: Functional status
	Secondary outcome: None
Number of centres	11
Stratification	GCS score

◆ Inclusion criteria: Age 16–65 years; non-penetrating head injury; GCS 3–8 post-resuscitation.

- Patients were excluded in the following circumstances: fixed pupils; poor resuscitation (low systolic BP, or poor oxygenation); non-neurological life-threatening injury; persistent medical condition; bleeding; pregnancy; delay in initiation of cooling.
- Target cooling temperature was 33°C (bladder) and was achieved with a combination of surface cooling, cold fluids, gastric lavage, and room air ventilation.
- Target temperature was aimed to be achieved within 8 h following injury.
- All patients had ICP monitoring.
- Analysis on an intention-to-treat basis.

Outcome measures

Primary endpoints

- Glasgow Outcome Scale (GOS): favourable outcome defined as good recovery or moderate disability; poor outcome defined as severe disability or worse at 6 months.

Other endpoints

- Neurobehavioural and neuropsychological tests at 6 months
- Deaths and complications also recorded

Results

The trial was stopped after 392 patients enrolled (199 to hypothermia arm, 193 to normo-thermia arm). Interim analysis had shown a probability of less than 0.01 of detecting a treatment effect if the trial was continued to target numbers of 500 patients.

	Hypothermia	Normothermia	Statistical significance
Poor outcome	57%	57%	None
Death	28%	27%	None

- In patients over the age of 45 there was a slightly higher percentage with poor outcome in the hypothermia group (88%) compared to the normothermia group (69%) but the difference was not statistically significant.
- No differences found in the two groups on neurobehavioural or neuropsychological testing.
- Patients who were hypothermic on admission who were randomized to the hypother-mic arm had 17% less poor outcomes than hypothermic patients randomized to the normothermia arm (not statistically significant).
- Although mean ICP was not affected by hypothermia there were statistically fewer patients with ICPs over 30 in the first 4 days.

Conclusions

Hypothermic treatment within 8 h following severe TBI does not improve functional outcome.

Critique

There are two hypothetical mechanisms by which hypothermia has been postulated to be beneficial in severe TBI: control of intracranial pressure rises; and a neuroprotective effect preventing secondary brain injury. This study by Clifton *et al.* is by far the largest study to date looking at the clinical effects of therapeutic hypothermia in severe TBI and has been called a landmark achievement for proving that it is ineffective (Narajan, 2001). It is of note that the trial was discontinued early due to lack of treatment effect. The authors also raised the possibility that there may even have been a detrimental effect of hypothermia in patients over the age of 45, although this was not statistically significant.

It has been suggested that there is a possibility that the results of the trial were affected by differences in fluid therapy and medication therapies between centres participating in the trial (Polderman *et al.*, 2001). Indeed, there was a statistically significant difference between the two treatment arms in terms of fluid balance, vasopressor therapy, and use of muscle relaxants. However, three separate meta-analyses of the available published trials support the conclusion that hypothermia is not beneficial in severe TBI (Harris *et al.*, 2002; Henderson *et al.*, 2003; McIntyre *et al.*, 2003).

Despite the negative result of the trial, several points were highlighted by the authors that suggest that questions still remain regarding the efficacy of hypothermia. For example, patients who were hypothermic on admission appeared to have a slightly better outcome (Clifton *et al.*, 2002). There may, therefore, be a role for ultra-early cooling of patients, perhaps even in the pre-hospital setting (Clifton, 2004). Also, none of the trials so far have addressed whether patient cooling to reduce raised intracranial pressure improves outcome (Clifton, 2004).

Following the study by Clifton *et al.*, the routine cooling of head-injured patients has been categorically determined to be ineffective. However, the study has revealed several avenues for further investigation regarding the use of hypothermia in severe TBI.

Clifton GL. Is keeping cool still hot? An update on hypothermia in brain injury. *Curr Opin Crit Care* 2004; **10**: 116–119.

Clifton GL, Miller E, Choi SC, Levin HS, McCauley S, Smith KRJ, Muizelaar JP, Marion DW, Luerssen TG. Hypothermia on admission in patients with severe brain injury. *J Neurotrauma* 2002; **19**: 293–301.

Harris OA, Colford JM, Good MC, Matx PG. The role of hypothermia in the management of severe brain injury. A meta-analysis. *Arch Neurol* 2002; **59**: 1077–1083.

Henderson WR, Dhingra VK, Chittock DR *et al.* Hypothermia in the management of traumatic brain injury. A systematic review and meta-analysis. *Intensive Care Med* 2003; **29**: 1637–1644.

McIntire LA, Fergusson DA, Herbert PC *et al.* Prolonged therapeutic hypothermia after traumatic brain injury in adults. *JAMA* 2003; **289**: 2992–2999.

Narajan RK. Hypothermia for traumatic brain injury – a good idea proved ineffective. *(Editorial) N Engl J Med* 2001; **344**: 602–603.

Polderman KH, Girbes ARJ, Peerdeman SM *et al.* Neurosurgical forum, letters to the editor. Hypothermia. *J Neurosurg* 2001; **94**: 853–855.

3.9 Hyperventilation in head injury

Details of study

The only randomized trial evaluating the role of hyperventilation on outcome in severe traumatic brain injury was (Muizelaar *et al.*, 1991) carried out at the Medical College of Virginia and was published in 1991. This trial has been the most influential study to date in indicating that prolonged hyperventilation should be avoided in severe traumatic brain injury. The trial compared normoventilation, hyperventilation, and hyperventilation plus tromomethamine (THAM). THAM was introduced to examine whether there was any effect of loss of CSF buffer during hyperventilation.

Study references

Main study

Muizelaar JP, Marmarou A, Ward JD, Kontos HA, Choi SC, Becker DP, Gruemer H, Young HF. Adverse effects of prolonged hyperventilation in patients with severe traumatic brain injury. *J Neurosurg* 1991; **75**: 731–739.

Related reference

Schierhout G, Roberts I. Hyperventilation therapy for acute traumatic brain injury. *Cochrane Database Syst Rev* 2000; (**2**):CD000566.

Study design

+ Randomized controlled trial

Class of evidence	II
Randomization	Normoventilation versus hyperventilation versus THAM
Number of patients	113
Follow-up	Primary outcomes: Glasgow Outcome Score at 3, 6, and 12 months
	Secondary outcomes: None
	100% follow-up
Number of centres	1
Stratification	On severity of head injury based on motor score of GCS (1–3 and 4–5)

+ Inclusion criteria: Age >3; GCS <9 following resuscitation and treatment of mass lesion.

+ In the normoventilation group, $Paco_2$ was kept in the range 30–35 mmHg for a period of 5 days.

+ In the hyperventilation groups, $Paco_2$ was kept in the 24–28 mmHg range for a period of 5 days.

+ THAM was administered as a bolus followed by a sustained intravenous infusion for 5 days.

Outcomes

Glasgow outcome scores were used and a favourable outcome was defined as a good outcome/moderate disability.

Results

The authors classified patients as having a favourable outcome if they were good or moderately disabled according to the GOS. Outcome results at 3 and 6 months for patients presenting with a GCS motor score 4–5.

	Favourable outcome		Statistical significance
	Normoventilation	Hyperventilation	
3 months	48%	18%	$p < 0.05$
6 months	57%	24%	$p < 0.05$

- There were no differences at 12 months follow-up.
- No differences were seen in the group with lower motor scores.

Conclusions

- Prophylactic hyperventilation is deleterious in head-injured patients who presented with a motor score of 4–5.
- The authors also concluded that the deleterious effect of sustained hyperventilation could be overcome by THAM.

Critique

Hyperventilation results in vasoconstriction induced by hypocarbia and effectively lowers ICP by reducing cerebral blood flow. Hyperventilation to rapidly reduce ICP has, therefore, long been employed in the management of TBI. However, there has always been concern that the reduction of cerebral blood flow itself could be deleterious due to resultant cerebral ischaemia. The authors of this study concluded that prolonged prophylactic hyperventilation is deleterious in head-injured patients. This study has been extremely influential as it has prompted recommendations that prolonged hyperventilation in TBI patients should be avoided because of potentially deleterious effects on outcome. However, this study has several weaknesses. Firstly, there was no blinding of the evaluator to the treatment received. Secondly, the majority of patients (86%) in this study did not have raised ICP on admission to hospital. Hyperventilation was, therefore, used prophylactically in this study, and it remains to be elucidated as to whether such measures to reduce ICP once it is elevated could be effective. Thirdly, there was no power calculation employed to determine the sample size required. Schierhout and Roberts concluded that the data from this trial were insufficient to determine whether hyperventilation is harmful or beneficial in TBI. Nonetheless, this study is the best study available to date examining the effects of hyperventilation. Further studies are required to examine what levels of $PaCO_2$ are optimal for the severe TBI patient and whether there is any role for either prolonged or transient hyperventilation to reduce elevated ICP in these patients.

Schierhout G, Roberts I. Hyperventilation therapy for acute traumatic brain injury. *Cochrane Database Syst Rev* 2000; (**2**):CD000566.

3.10 **Magnesium for neuroprotection in head injury**

Details of study

The study by Temkin *et al.* (2007) set out to determine whether there is any benefit from magnesium sulphate infusions in preventing secondary brain injury in patients with TBI. The study was carried out at the Haborview Medical Center in Seattle, USA, over a 6-year period between 1998 and 2004.

Study references

Main study

Temkin NR, Anderson GD, Winn HR, Ellenbagen RG, Schuster J, Lucas T, Newell DW, Mansfield PN, Machamer JE, Barber J, Dikmen SS. Magnesium sulfate for neuroprotection after traumatic brain injury: a randomised controlled trial. *Lancet Neurol* 2007; **6**: 29–38.

Related reference

Muir KW, Lees KR, Ford I, Davis S. Magnesium for acute stroke (Intravenous Magnesium Efficacy in Stroke trial): a randomised controlled trial. *Lancet* 2004; **363**: 439–445.

Study design

* Double-blind, parallel group, randomized trial
* A Phase III trial

Class of evidence	II
Randomization	Magnesium versus placebo
Number of patients	499
Follow-up	6 months
	Primary outcomes: Functional status, seizures, neuropsychological tests
	Secondary outcome: None
Number of centres	1
Stratification	Severity of injury Age of patient

* IV MgSO$_4$ (or saline placebo) given within 8 h of injury and continued for 5 days.
* Target plasma concentration was initially high 1.25–2.5 mmol/L but this was adjusted later to a lower level of 1.0–1.8 mmol/L.
* Patients with hypomagnesia had their magnesium levels corrected.
* Moderate TBI defined as: GCS 9–12 (or motor score 4–5).
* Severe TBI defined as: 3–8 (or motor score 1–3), or need for intracranial surgery.

- Patients excluded if <14 years of age, pregnant, or delay in receiving infusion.
- Analysis on intention-to-treat basis.

Outcome measures

Primary endpoints

- Survival time
- Functional outcome at 6 months: GOSE
- Seizures—time to early (<1 week post injury) or late (>1 week post injury)
- Neuropsychological tests of attention, information processing, memory, and intellectual function
- All endpoints analysed at 6 months although some, e.g. GOSE, assessed at 1 and 3 months also

Secondary endpoints

- None

Results

- 93% follow-up at 6 months.
- Primary outcomes were analysed as a composite and no positive effect for $MgSO_4$ found.
- Blood pressure was lower in the $MgSO_4$ treated group for the higher serum levels but not for the lower target levels.

Outcome	High $MgSO_4$			Low $MgSO_4$		
	$MgSO_4$	Placebo	Stat. Sig.	$MgSO_4$	Placebo	Statistical significance
Mortality	28%	14%	$p = 0.05$	24%	20%	None
Late seizures	17%	13%	$p = 0.05$	9%	6%	None
GOSE	57	54	None	176	174	None

- GOSE of >5 (moderate disability or better) was 49% for high-dose $MgSO_4$ versus 40% for placebo and 38% for low-dose $MgSO_4$ versus 42% for placebo.

Conclusions

Intravenous $MgSO_4$ given within 8 h of moderate to severe TBI does not improve outcome and may even have a detrimental effect.

Critique

Although the study was carried out at a single centre, the authors have argued that it was a regional level I trauma unit for a whole state and so it is appropriate to generalize from their results. However, the power of the trial would undoubtedly be increased by the inclusion of more than one study centre.

The use of a composite primary outcome is an interesting method to increase power of trial and the authors have been commended for this novel approach. It has been standard practice to dichotomize patient outcome into favourable or unfavourable on the basis of the GOSE score. Proponents of composite analysis argue that dichotomizing outcome may be insensitive. However, the authors of this trial have been criticized for using 39 outcome measures to be included in their composite analysis, which may be too many (Maas and Murray, 2007). Freemantle *et al.* have reviewed the arguments for and against the use of composite outcomes in clinical trials (Freemantle *et al.*, 2005).

One of the most crucial points that needs to be emphasized when interpreting the results of this trial is that it was restarted with a lower target $MgSO_4$ concentration and that analysis of the two target levels was carried out separately. This has been questioned as to whether an analysis of the two groups together would have given rise to more drug-specific conclusions (Maas and Murray, 2007). As things stand, conclusions can only be made regarding specific dosing regimes. Nonetheless, the timing and target ranges used in the trial are consistent with those that have been widely used in the management of head injury. It is legitimate for the authors, therefore, to draw the conclusion that there is no evidence for a beneficial effect of standard methods of $MgSO_4$ infusions in head injury.

Following this trial there is currently no evidence to support the use of magnesium sulphate infusions as a neuroprotective measure in head injury. In addition, the novel use of a composite analysis may influence the design and outcome assessment of future head-injury trials.

Freemantle N, Calvert M, Wood J, Eastaugh J, Griffin C. Composite outcomes in randomised trials: greater precision but with greater uncertainty. *JAMA* 2005; **289**: 2554–2559.

Maas AIR, Murray GD. Magnesium for neuroprotection after traumatic brain injury. *Lancet Neurol* 2007; **6**: 20–21.

3.11 Epidemiology of post-traumatic seizures

Details of studies

Two large population-based studies looking at the epidemiology of PTS stand out as landmarks in elucidating the epidemiology of post-traumatic seizures in traumatic brain injury. The first study included 4541 people who suffered traumatic brain injuries over a 50-year period (1935–1984) in Olmsted County, Minnesota, USA (Annegers *et al.*, 1998). The second study followed 78,572 people with TBI born over a 25-year period (1977–2002) in Denmark (Christensen *et al.*, 2009).

Study references

Main studies

Annegers JF, Hauser WA, Coan SP, Rocca WA. A population-based study of seizures after traumatic brain injuries. *N Engl J Med* 1998; **338**: 20–24.

Christensen J, Pedersen MG, Pedersen CB, Sidenius P, Olsen J, Vestergaard M. Long-term risk of epilepsy after traumatic brain injury in children and young adults: a population-based cohort study. *Lancet* 2009; **373**: 1105–1110.

Related references

Englander J, Bushnik T, Duong TT, Cifu DX, Zafonte R, Wright J, Hughes R, Bergman W. Analyzing risk factors for late posttraumatic seizures: a prospective, multicenter investigation. *Arch Phys Med Rehabil* 2003; **83**: 365–373.

Salazar AM, Jabbari B, Vance SC, Grafman J, Amin D, Dillon JD. Epilepsy after penetrating head injury. I. Clinical correlates: a report of the Vietnam Head Injury Study. *Neurology* 1985; **35**: 1406–1414.

Temkin NR. Risk factors for posttraumatic seizures in adults. *Epilepsia* 2003; **44**: 18–20.

Study design

Annegers *et al.*

This was a population-based study that used an epidemiology database to identify diagnoses of TBI over a 50-year period and then followed the patients up to identify occurrence of seizures. Patients were excluded if the TBI was fatal, if they had pre-existing epilepsy, or if they suffered subsequent TBI. TBI was divided into three categories:

Mild TBI	◆ No skull fracture ◆ Loss of consciousness or post-traumatic amnesia < 30 min
Moderate TBI	≥1 of the following: ◆ Loss of consciousness or post-traumatic amnesia > 30 min but <24 h ◆ Skull fracture
Severe TBI	≥1 of the following: ◆ Contusion ◆ Intracranial haematoma ◆ Loss of consciousness or post-traumatic amnesia > 24 h

Christensen *et al.*

This was a population-based study that used the Civil Registration System in Denmark to identify 1,605,216 people born between 1977 and 2002, which amounted to a total of

19,527,337 person-years. Relative risk (RR) of epilepsy was calculated for mild brain injury, severe brain injury, and skull fracture. Time since injury and variables of age, sex, and family history of epilepsy were considered. Definition of mild and severe brain injury were according to the American Congress of Rehabilitation Medicine: mild brain injury is manifest by altered brain function (loss of consciousness <30 min, GCS not less than 13, amnesia <24 h, confusion); severe brain injury includes contusion and intracranial haemorrhage.

Results

Annegers *et al.*

Severity of TBI	Cumulative 5-year probability of seizure	Standardized incidence ratio
Mild	0.7%	1.5
Moderate	1.2%	2.9
Severe	10.0%	17.0

- There was no increased risk of seizures for mild TBI after 5 years.
- Patients with moderate TBI retain a significantly increased risk of seizures for over 10 years.
- Patients with severe TBI retained a significantly increased risk of seizures for over 20 years.
- Strongest risk factors for PTS: brain contusions and subdural haematomas.
- Other risk factors for PTS: skull fracture and prolonged loss of consciousness.

Christensen *et al.*

	Relative risk of epilepsy after head injury	Relative risk of epilepsy > 10 years after head injury
Mild head injury	2.22	1.51
Moderate head injury	7.40	4.29
Skull fracture	2.17	2.06

- RR of epilepsy increased with age, and in patients >15 years of age at time of injury RR was 3.51 for mild and 12.24 for severe head injury.
- RR of epilepsy was higher in women (2.49) compared to men (2.01).
- RR of epilepsy was also increased in those with a family history of epilepsy (5.75 mild and 10.09 severe head injury).

Conclusions

Annegers *et al.*

The risk of PTS increases with the severity of the TBI and varies according to the time since the injury.

Christensen *et al.*

Traumatic head injury is a long-lasting risk factor for epilepsy and there is a window for prevention of post-traumatic epilepsy.

Critique

These two studies are the largest and best population-based studies concerning the epidemiology of post-traumatic epilepsy available. The study by Annegers *et al.* gave valuable data regarding the duration of risk of PTS and the relation of severity of injury to this increased risk. The authors also identified several factors, such as subdural haematoma and brain contusions, which increase the risk of PTS. However, the study by Christensen *et al.* found that the risk of epilepsy following TBI remains high for far longer than 5 years, and in their study was still present at >10 years following injury. However, this difference may reflect the wider inclusion criteria of the Danish study or the smaller sample size of the US study. The Danish study has been criticized for not evaluating the type of seizures or the timing of the seizures, e.g. early or late (Shorvon and Neligan, 2009). Furthermore, there were no details regarding whether the dura was breached nor in those patients with skull fractures. Another criticism is that the data collection only included outpatient follow-up since 1995 and it is possible that many seizures will have been diagonsed in this setting. Nonetheless, both studies included here provide the best epidemiological data avialable for elucidating the risk of post-traumatic epilepsy.

Shorvon S, Neligan A. Risk of epilespy after head trauma. *Lancet* 2009; **373**: 1060–1061.

3.12 **Phenytoin for prevention of post-traumatic seizures**

Details of study

This study (Temkin *et al.*, 1990) was the first PRCT deemed to have sufficient power to evaluate the efficacy of phenytoin for the prophylaxis of PTS following serious head injury. The study was carried out in the mid-1980s at the Harborview Medical Center, Seattle, Washington, USA.

Study references

Main study

Temkin NR, Dikmen SS, Wilensky AJ, Keihm J, Chabal S, Winn HR. A randomised, double-blind study of phenytoin for the prevention of post-traumatic seizures. *N Engl J Med* 1990; **323**: 497–502.

Related references

Annegers JF, Hauser WA, Coan SP, Rocca WA. A population-based study of seizures after traumatic brain injuries. *N Engl J Med* 1998; **338**: 20–24.

Schierhout G, Roberts I. Anti-epileptic drugs for preventing seizures following acute traumatic brain injury. *Cochrane Database Syst Rev* 2001; **4**: CD000173.

Study design

• Double-blind PRCT

Class of evidence	I
Randomization	Phenytoin versus placebo
Number of patients	404
Follow-up	Primary outcomes: Early seizures (1st week)
	Secondary outcomes: Late seizures (1 week to 24 months)
	Percentage of patients followed up at each stage? (> 80%?)
Number of centres	1
Stratification	None

• Patients were included if: Presence of a severe head injury defined as one or more of: cortical contusion (visible on CT scan); subdural haematoma (SDH); EDH; ICH; depressed skull fracture; penetrating head injury; seizure <24 h from injury; GCS ≤ 10).

• Patients were excluded if they were <16 years old or there was a delay of > 24 h before loading of drug.

• Patients were also excluded if there were other predisposing risk factors for seizures, e.g. previous severe head injury, history of severe alcoholism, or previous neurological conditions with risk of seizures.

- Initial loading dose of phenytoin was 20 mg/kg with maintenance dose adjusted according to serum levels.
- Phenytoin/placebo continued for 12 months and was then tapered off fully.
- Analysis was on an intention-to-treat basis.

Outcome measures

Primary endpoints

- The occurrence of seizures: early (<1 week); or late (>1 week)
- Diagnosis of seizures by experienced clinician with the use of EEG recording if required

Other endpoints analysed

- Possible adverse effects of phenytoin

Results

Outcome	Phenytoin group	Placebo group	Statistical significance
Early seizure rate (cumulative)	3.6 ± 1.3%	14.2 ± 2.6%	$p < 0.001$
Late seizure rate (2 years)	27.5 ± 4.0%	21.1 ± 3.7%	None

- Phenytoin treatment reduced risk of seizures by 73% in the first week.
- Additional secondary analysis revealed no difference in the cumulative probability of all seizures (early or late) in both groups.

Conclusions

Phenytoin has a beneficial effect in reducing the incidence of post-traumatic seizures only in the first week following severe head injury.

Critique

Although previous RCT had been carried out, this study may be regarded as the first PRCT with sufficient numbers of patients recruited to analyse the efficacy of phenytoin for the prophylaxis of post-traumatic seizures. Meta-analysis of all published trials supports the findings of this study. A Cochrane review in 2001 identified six published randomized controlled trials looking at seizure prophylaxis for post-traumatic epilepsy and concluded that the use of anticonvulsants would keep 1 in 10 patients seizure free in the first week following head injury but that there was no evidence for efficacy against late seizures (Schierhout and Roberts, 2001).

Schierhout G, Roberts I. Anti-epileptic drugs for preventing seizures following acute traumatic brain injury. *Cochrane Database Syst Rev* 2001; 4: CD000173.

Chapter 4

Spinal surgery

RD Johnson, JCD Leach, WA Liebenberg,
N Maartens, SA Cudlip

4.0 **Introduction**

The field of spinal surgery is shared by both neurosurgeons and spinal orthopaedic surgeons. Over the last few decades improved spinal imaging modalities have become widely available in the form of computed tomography (CT) and magnetic resonance imaging (MRI). This has allowed for better correlation of clinical, radiological, and surgical findings. The classic dilemmas and controversies that have faced spinal surgery in the past are, therefore, being revisited in this era of neuroimaging. Searching an online database with the terms 'spinal surgery' and 'clinical trial' will bring up hundreds, if not thousands, of results. This also reflects the advent of a myriad of new spinal adjuncts and prostheses that are making their way into the spinal surgeon's tool box. In this chapter, we have endeavoured to steer away from studies that compare spinal prosthetics or fusion devices and concentrate rather on the core aspects of spinal practice that is relevant to most neurosurgeons. We have, therefore, included studies that address the role of decompressive surgery in the management of spine or nerve root compression whether this may be from trauma, degenerative disease, or tumours. This approach has allowed us to include trials looking at the role of steroids in the management of spinal cord compression secondary to trauma and metastatic disease (Bracken *et al.*, 1984; Bracken *et al.*, 1985; Vecht *et al*, 1989; Bracken *et al.*, 1990; Bracken *et al.*, 1997). In addition, we have included studies on the role of surgical decompression in the management of cord compression secondary to trauma and metastatic disease (Vaccaro *et al.*, 1997; Patchell *et al.*, 2005). Several studies have been included that address the role of surgery in lumbar disc prolapse including the results of the recently reported Spine Patient Outcomes Research Trial (SPORT) in the United States (Weber, 1983; Weinstein, *et al.*, 2006; Barth *et al.*, 2008a; Barth *et al.*, 2008b; Peul *et al.*, 2008). Included here is a section on the timing of surgery for cauda equine syndrome (CES) (O'Laoire *et al.*, 1981). This is a highly contentious area and although there is no randomized trial there are two meta-analyses that have provoked considerable discussion and debate in the literature (Ahn *et al.*, 2000; Todd, 2005). The role of surgery in the management of lumbar stenosis was also examined as part of the SPORT trial and so we have included it here for completion (Weinstein *et al.*, 2007). This large trial demonstrates many of the difficulties in conducting trials in spinal patients. The Medical Research Council (MRC) trial on the role of spinal stabilization surgery in chronic back pain has also been included in this section (Fairbank *et al.*, 2005). There are numerous case series and evidence-based reviews of different aspects of cervical spine surgery including randomized studies evaluating the efficacy of different spinal implants. However, we have chosen to include here two prospective randomized studies that compare surgery with conservative measures for the treatment of cervical myelopathy and cervical radiculopathy.

Ahn UM, Ahn NU, Buchowski MS, Garrett ES, Sieber AN, Kostuik JP. Cauda equina syndrome secondary to lumbar disc herniation. A meta-analysis of surgical outcomes. *Spine* 2000; **25**: 1515–1522.

Barth M, Diepers M, Weiss C, Thome C. Two-year outcome after lumbar microdiscectomy versus microscopic sequestrectomy: part1: evaluation of clinical outcome. *Spine* 2008a; **33**: 265–272.

Barth M, Diepers M, Weiss C, Thome C. Two-year outcome after lumbar microdiscectomy versus microscopic sequestrectomy: part 2: radiographic evaluation and correlation with clinical outcome. *Spine* 2008b; **33**: 273–279.

Bracken MB, Collings WF, Freeman DF, Shepard MJ, Wagner FW, Silten RM, *et al.* Efficacy of methyl-prednisolone in acute spinal cord injury. *JAMA* 1984; **251**: 45–52.

Bracken MB, Shepard MJ, Hellenbrand KG, Collins WF, Leo LS, Freeman DF, Wagner FC, Flamm ES, Eisenberg HM, Goodman JH, *et al.* Methylprednisolone and neurological function 1 year after spinal cord injury. Results of the National Acute Spinal Cord Injury Study. *J Neurosurg* 1985; **63**: 704–713.

Bracken MB, Shepard MJ, Collins WF, Holford TR, Young W, Baskin DS, Eisenberg HM, Flamm E, Leo-Summers L, Maroon J, *et al.* A randomized, controlled trial of methylprednisolone or naloxone in the treatment of acute spinal-cord injury. Results of the Second National Acute Spinal Cord Injury Study. *N Engl J Med* 1990; **322**: 1405–1411.

Bracken MB, Shepard MJ, Holford TR, Leo-Summers L, Aldrich EF, Fazl M, Fehlings M, Herr DL, Hitchon PW, Marshall LF, Nockels RP, Pascale V, Perot PL Jr, Piepmeier J, Sonntag VK, Wagner F, Wilberger JE, Winn HR, Young W. Administration of methylprednisolone for 24 or 48 hours or tirilazad mesylate for 48 hours in the treatment of acute spinal cord injury. Results of the Third National Acute Spinal Cord Injury Randomized Controlled Trial. National Acute Spinal Cord Injury Study. *JAMA* 1997; **277**: 1597–1604.

Fairbank J, Frost H, Wilson-MacDonald J, Yu LM, Barker K, Collins R for the Spine Stabilisation Trial Group. Randomised controlled trial to compare surgical stabilisation of the lumbar spine with an intensive rehabilitation programme for patients with chronic low back pain: the MRC spine stabilisation trial. *BMJ* 2005; **330**: 1233–1240.

O'Laoire SA, Crockard HA, Thomas DG. Prognosis for sphinctor recovery after operation for operaton for cauda equina compression owing to lumbar disc prolapse. *BMJ* 1981; **282**: 1852–1854.

Patchell RA, Tibbs PA, Regine WF, Saris S, Kryscio RJ, Mohiuddin M, Young B. Direct decompressive surgical resection in the treatment of spinal cord compression caused by metastatic cancer. *Lancet* 2005; **366**: 643–648.

Peul WC, van den Hout WB, Brand R, Thomeer RTWM, Koes BW, for the Leiden – The Hague Spine Intervention Prognostic Study Group. Prolonged conservative care versus early surgery in patients with sciatica caused by lumbar disc herniation: two year results of a randomised controlled trial. *BMJ* 2008; **336**: 1355–1358.

SPORT trial – several things looked at but reported separately, so covered here in its separate entities.

Tator CH, Fehlings MG, Thorpe K, Taylor W. Current use and timing of spinal surgery for management of acute spinal surgery for management of acute spinal cord injury in North America: results of a retrospective multicenter study. *J Neurosurg* 1999; **91**: 12–18.

Todd NV. Cauda equina syndrome: the timing of surgery probably does influence outcome. *B J Neurosurg* 2005; **19**: 301–306.

Vaccaro AR, Daugherty RJ, Sheehan J, Sheehan TP, Dante SJ, Cotle JM, Ba derston RA, Herbison GJ, Northup BE. Neurologic outcome of early versus later surgery for cervical cord injury. *Spine* 1997; **22**: 2609–2613.

Vecht CJ, Haaxma-Reiche H, van Putten WL, de Visser M, Vries EP, Twiijnstra A. Initial bolus of conventional versus high-dose dexamethasone in metastatic spinal cord compression. *Neurology* 1989; **39**: 1255–1257.

Weber H. Lumbar disc herniation. A controlled, prospective study with ten years of observation. *Spine* 1983; **8**: 131–140.

Weinstein JN, Tosteson TD, Lurie JD, Tosteson ANA, Hnascom B, Skinner JS, Abdu WA, Hilibrand AS, Boden SD, Deyo RA. Surgical vs nonoperative treatment of lumbar disk herniation: the spine patient outcomes research trial (SPORT): a randomised trial. *JAMA* 2006; **296**: 2441–2450.

Weinstein JN, Lurie JD, Tosteson TD, Hanscom B, Tosteson ANA, Blood EA, Birkmeyer NJO, Hilibrand AS, Herkowitz H, Cammisa FP, Todd JA, Emery SE, Lenke LG, Abdu WA, Longley M, Errico TJ, Hu SS. Surgery versus nonsurgical treatment for lumbar degenerative spondylolisthesis. *New Engl J Med* 2007; **356**: 2257–2270.

Weinstein JN, Tosteson TD, Lurie JD, Tosteson ANA, Blood E, Hanscom B, Herkwoitz H, Cammisa F, Albert T, Boden SD, Hilibrand A, Goldberg H, Berven S, An H for the SPORT Investigators. Surgical versus nonsurgical therapy for lumbar spinal stenosis. *N Engl J Med* 2008; **358**: 794–810.

4.1 **Steroids for acute spinal cord injury**

Details of study

The National Acute Spinal Cord Injury Study (NASCIS) is the largest study investigating the effects of the steroid methyl prednisolone (MePred) in acute spinal cord injury. There have been three parts to the study that are referred to as NASCIS I, NASCIS II, and NASCIS III. These studies were carried out in the United States in the 1980s and 1990s.

Study references

Main study

There are four main references for the NASCIS study:

Bracken MB, Collings WF, Freeman DF, Shepard MJ, Wagner FW, Silten RM *et al*. Efficacy of methyl-prednisolone in acute spinal cord injury. *JAMA* 1984; **251**: 45–52.

Bracken MB, Shepard MJ, Hellenbrand KG, Collins WF, Leo LS, Freeman DF, Wagner FC, Flamm ES, Eisenberg HM, Goodman JH, *et al*. Methylprednisolone and neurological function 1 year after spinal cord injury. Results of the National Acute Spinal Cord Injury Study. *J Neurosurg* 1985; **63**: 704–713.

Bracken MB, Shepard MJ, Collins WF, Holford TR, Young W, Baskin DS, Eisenberg HM, Flamm E, Leo-Summers L, Maroon J, *et al*. A randomized, controlled trial of methylprednisolone or naloxone in the treatment of acute spinal-cord injury. Results of the Second National Acute Spinal Cord Injury Study. *N Engl J Med* 1990; **322**: 1405–1411

Bracken MB, Shepard MJ, Holford TR, Leo-Summers L, Aldrich EF, Fazl M, Fehlings M, Herr DL, Hitchon PW, Marshall LF, Nockels RP, Pascale V, Perot PL Jr, Piepmeier J, Sonntag VK, Wagner F, Wilberger JE, Winn HR, Young W. Administration of methylprednisolone for 24 or 48 hours or tirilazad mesylate for 48 hours in the treatment of acute spinal cord injury. Results of the Third National Acute Spinal Cord Injury Randomized Controlled Trial. National Acute Spinal Cord Injury Study. *JAMA* 1997; **277**: 1597–1604.

Related references

Bracken MB. Steroids for acute spinal cord injury. Cochrane Database of Syst Rev 2002; **3**: CD001046.

Otani K, Abe H, Kadoya K, *et al*. Beneficial effect of methylprednisolone sodium citrate in the treatment of acute spinal cord injury. *Sekitui Skeizui J* 1994; **7**: 633–647.

Petijean ME, Pontillart V, Dixmarias F, Wiart K, Sztark F, Lassie P, Thicoipe M, Dabadie P. Traitement medicamenteux de la lesion medullaire traumatique au stade aigu. *Ann Fr Aneth Reanim* 1998; **17**: 115–122.

Study design

♦ Multi-centre, blinded, PRCTs

	NASCIS I	NASCIS II	NASCIS III
Class of evidence	I	I	I
Randomization	Moderate-dose versus low-dose MePred	MePred versus naloxone versus placebo	24 h MePred versus 48 h MePred versus 48 h tirilazad mesylate
Number of patients	330	487	499

	NASCIS I	NASCIS II	NASCIS III
Follow-up	6 weeks, 6 months, 1 year	6 weeks, 6 months, 1 year	6 weeks, 6 months, 1 year
	Primary outcomes: Neurological status, morbidity, and mortality	Primary outcomes: Neurological status, morbidity, and mortality	Primary outcomes: Neurological status, morbidity, and mortality
	Secondary: None	Secondary: None	Secondary: None
Number of Centres	9	10	16
Stratification	Neurological status at time of injury	1 Early versus late treatment with steroid 2 Complete or incomplete cord injury	Ultra-early versus early treatment with steroid

Dosing

- NASCIS I: low-dose regimen—loading dose of MePred was 100 mg followed by 25 mg every 6 h for 10 days; moderate-dose regimen—1000 mg bolus followed by 250 mg every 6 h for 10 days.
- NASCIS II: MePred was given as an intravenous bolus of 30 mg/kg followed by 5.4 mg/kg for 23 h.
- NASCIS III: MePred bolus and maintenance infusions given as per NASCIS II except continued for further 23 or 47 h.

Timing of bolus

- NASCIS II looked at early (<8 h from injury) versus late (>8 h) administration of MePred.
- NASCIS III also looked at ultra-early (<3 h) versus early (3–8 h) administration of MePred.

Outcome measures

Primary endpoints

- Neurological status was measured on continuous numerical scales in a blinded manner, e.g. muscle function was measured in 14 muscle segments on a 6-point scale between 0 and 5 (total score 70).

Results

NASCIS I

- There was no difference between moderate-dose and low-dose MePred.
- There was a trend towards better outcome for moderate-dose MePred if given within 8 h.

NASCIS II

- Patients who received MePred within 8 h of injury had a statistically significant improvement in motor and sensory function.
- There was no effect of naloxone.

NASCIS III

- No statistically significant benefit was seen for continuing MePred treatment for 48 h.
- No statistically significant benefit was seen for ultra-early administration of MePred.

Conclusions

MePred improves outcome of acute spinal cord injury (ASCI) if given within 8 h of injury.

Critique

The positive results of the NASCIS trials pertain only to post-hoc subgroup analyses. For example, NASCIS II only showed a benefit with MePred for the subgroup of patients who received it within 8 h of injury. It is imperative, therefore, to re-emphasize that the conclusions from this subgroup analysis cannot be extended to all patients within the trial. The large range of the neurological scores used has meant that it is questionable whether small improvements are clinically relevant (Spencer and Bazarian, 2003).

Spinal cord injury is a devastating disorder with approximately 10% mortality and high rates of severe disability. NASCIS I is probably the first clinical trial of a therapeutic intervention in acute spinal cord injury. Together the three NASCIS trials form the largest study to date looking at the effects of steroids in ASCI. However, the results remain controversial and there is as yet no guideline or recommendations regarding the use of steroids in ASCI. The use of MePred is, therefore, still a treatment choice available to the managing surgeon.

Coleman WP, Benzel D, Cahill DW, Ducker T, Geisler F, Green B, *et al.* A critical appraisal of the reporting of the National Acute Spinal Cord Injury Studies (II and III) of methylprednisolone in acute spinal cord injury. *J Spinal Disord* 2000; **13**: 185–199.

Hubert RJ. Methylprednisolone for acute spinal cord injury: an inappropriate standard of care. *J Neurosurg* 2000; **93**: S1–S7.

Spencer MT, Bazarian JJ. Are corticosteroids effective in traumatic spinal cord injury? *Ann Emerg Med* 2003; **41**: 410–413.

4.2 **Steroids for metastatic spinal cord compression**

Details of Study

A blinded randomized controlled trial of high-dose dexamethasone as an adjunct to radiotherapy in patients with metastatic spinal cord compression (MESCC) from solid tumours was carried out between 1987 and 1989 in Rigshospitalet, Copenhagen, Denmark (Sorensen *et al.*, 1994).

Study references

Main study

Sorensen PS, Helwig-Larson S, Mouridesen H Hansen HH. Effect of high-dose dexamethasone in carcinomatous metastatic spinal cord compression treated with radiotherapy: a randomized trial. *Eur J Cancer* 1994; **30A**: 22–27

Related reference

Sciubba DM, Gokaslan ZL. Diagnosis and management of metastatic spine disease. *Surgical Oncology* 2006; **15**: 141–151.

Study design

* A single-blind PRCT

Class of evidence	II
Randomization	High-dose dexamethasone versus no steroids
Number of patients	57
Follow-up	6 months
	Primary outcomes: Preservation or return of gait function
	Secondary outcomes: Side effects Survival
Number of centres	1
Stratification	Primary tumour Gait function

* Dexamethasone was administered as a bolus of 96 mg IV followed by 96 mg PO for 3 days.
* Inclusion criteria: Clinical and radiological evidence of metastatic spinal cord compression.
* Exclusion criteria: Lymphoma patients; surgical decompression; previous epidural metastases; meningeal carcinomatosis; peptic ulcers.
* Analysis was done on an intention-to-treat basis.

Outcomes

Primary outcome

* Gait function

- Successful treatment was defined as walking ability retained (ambulatory patients) or walking ability regained (non-ambulatory patients).
- The same neurologist assessed all patients at 3 weeks after treatment and then 3-monthly until 2 years, or until patient deceased.

Results

- Follow-up 2 years (or until death).

	Dexamethasone	No steroids	Statistical significance
Return of gait function at 3 months	81%	63%	None
Percentage ambulatory at 6 months	59%	33%	$p = 0.05$

- There was no difference in survival between the two groups.
- Eleven percent of those receiving steroids experienced side effects.
- A subgroup analysis was carried out in patients with breast cancer, which showed that 94% of patients receiving dexamethasone achieved a successful result compared to 69% receiving no steroids. This result was not statistically significant.

Conclusion

Steroids should be administered routinely to all patients with MESCC.

Critique

Metastatic malignant cord compression is one of the most devastating and dreaded complications of cancer. Rapid neurological deterioration can result in paralysis and loss of sphincter function. The early diagnosis and treatment of this condition involves close cooperation between oncologists and neurosurgeons. Steroids are part of the treatment armamentarium available to try and reduce the incidence of severe neurological deficits in this condition.

This study by Sorensen et al. was the first randomized trial to examine the efficacy of steroids for MESCC. Prior to 1993 there was only a plethora of anecdotal reports regarding the benefits of steroids in this condition. The first report published in the late 1960s was of two patients with disseminated pelvic malignancies whose paraparesis improved following the administration of MePred (Cantu, 1968). Clarke and Saunders reported improvement in limb neurology in two children who were given steroids for a presumptive diagnosis of Guillain–Barré syndrome: both patients were subsequently found to have malignant cord compression (Clarke and Saunders, 1975). These observations of a beneficial effect of steroids were confirmed in animal models of malignant cord compression (Ushio et al., 1977). This led to the development of dosing regimens and protocols for the use in patients (Gilbert et al., 1978; Greenberg et al., 1980). The study by Sorenson et al.

followed on from this work. Although the benefit reached only borderline statistical significance the authors concluded that steroids should be used as an adjunct in malignant cord compression. This study established the role of steroids in this devastating condition.

Cantu RC. Corticosteroids for spinal metastases. *Lancet* 1968; **2**: 912.

Clarke PR, Saunders M. Steroid-induced remission in spinal canal reticulum cell sarcoma. Report of two cases. *J Neurosurg* 1975; **42**: 346–413.

Gilbert RW, Kim JH, Posner JB. Epidural spinal cord compression from metastatic tumor: diagnosis and treatment. *Ann Neurol* 1978; **3**: 40–51.

Greenberg HS, Kim JH, Posner JB. Epidural spinal cord compression from metastatic tumor: results with a new treatment protocol. *Ann Neurol* 1980; **8**: 361–366.

Ushio Y, Posner R, Posner JB, Shapiro WR. Experimental spinal cord compression by epidural neoplasm. *Neurology* 1977; **27**: 422–429.

4.3 Timing of surgery for acute spinal cord injury

Details of study

Most studies on the timing of surgery in acute spinal cord injury are either retrospective or prospective case series. This study undertaken at the Regional Spinal Cord Injury Center of Delaware Valley between 1992 and 1995 is the only attempt at a randomized controlled trial of surgery for acute spinal cord injury.

Study references

Main study

Vaccaro AR, Daugherty RJ, Sheehan J, Sheehan TP, Dante SJ, Cotle JM, Balsderston, RA, Herbison GJ, Northup BE. Neurologic outcome of early versus later surgery for cervical cord injury. *Spine* 1997; **22**: 2609–2613.

Related references

Bagnall AM, Jones L, Duffy S, Riemsma RP. Spinal fixation surgery for acute traumatic spinal cord injury. *Cochrane Database Syst Rev* 2008: CD004725.

Fehlings MG, Perrin RG. The role and timing of early decompression for cervical spinal cord injury: update with a review of recent clinical evidence. *Injury* 2005; **36**: SB13–SB26.

Fehlings MG, Perrin RG. The timing of surgical intervention in the treatment of spinal cord injury: a systematic review of recent clinical evidence. *Spine* 2006; **31**: 528–535.

Tator CH, Fehlings MG, Thorpe K, Taylor W. Current use and timing of spinal surgery for management of acute spinal cord injury in North America: results of a retrospective multicenter study. *J Neurosurg* 1999; **91**: 12–18.

Study design

- PRCT

Class of evidence	II
Randomization	Early surgery versus late surgery for cervical spinal cord trauma
Number of patients	64 randomized
Follow-up	< 1 year
	Primary outcomes: Neurologic outcome Functional outcome
	Secondary outcomes: Length of hospital stay
Number of centres	1
Stratification	Age and sex

- Inclusion criteria: Age 15–75 years; neurologic impairment A–D on American Spinal Injury Association (ASIA) scale; neurologic level C3–T1; admission within 48 h of injury; radiological evidence of cord compression.

- Exclusion criteria: Other injuries preventing neurological evaluation or surgery; coexisting spinal cord disease; worsening neurology due to blood, disc or bony fragments within the canal.
- Early surgery was <72 h from injury.
- Late surgery was >5 days from injury.
- Surgery included decompression ± stabilization procedures.
- Neurological outcome was assessed by comparing standard neurological examination before (on admission) and after surgery (mean 300 days).

Results

- Mean time to surgery was 1.8 days in the early group and 16.8 days in the late group.
- There were no significant differences in the neurological or functional outcomes between the two groups, or in the length of hospital stay.

Conclusions

There is no benefit between surgery within 72 h of injury and delayed surgery in cervical spinal cord injury.

Critique

The study by Vaccaro *et al.* includes only cases of cervical cord injury and the length of time to early surgery (mean 1.8 days) may not be early enough. It is still possible that there may be a benefit of earlier surgery within 8 or 12 h of injury. Tator *et al.* reported one of the largest case series in the literature looking at the effect of timing of surgery on outcome in ASCI at all spinal levels (Tator *et al.*, 1999). They conducted a retrospective analysis of over 500 cases of acute spinal cord injury admitted to 36 centres in North America over a period of 9 months. The results suggested that there is no agreement on the timing of surgery for ASCI and that further randomized controlled trials are needed. To date, the study by Vaccaro *et al.* remains the only attempt at a randomized trial. Fehlings and Perrin have published several comprehensive reviews of the literature on the timing of surgery in ASCI (Fehlings and Perrin, 2005; Fehlings and Perrin, 2006). On the basis of the published data, they have made recommendations regarding the timing of surgery in ASCI. However, they emphasize that with the lack of definitive evidence urgent decompression remains only a reasonable practice option that can be carried out safely.

4.4 **Decompressive surgery for spinal metastasis**

Details of study

This multi-instituitional study is the largest randomized study looking at the role of decompressive surgery in the management of metastatic spinal cord compression (MESCC). The study was carried out by the Bluegrass Neuro-Oncology Consortium in the United States.

Study references

Main study

Patchell RA, Tibbs PA, Regine WF, Payne R, Saris S, Kryscio RJ, Mohiuddin M, Young B. Direct decompressive surgical resection in the treatment of spinal cord compression caused by metastatic cancer: a randomised trial. *Lancet* 2005; **366**: 643–648.

Related reference

Ibrahim A, Crockard A, Antonietti P, Boriani S, Bunger C, Gasbarrini A, Grejes A, Harms J, Kawahara N, Mazel C, Melcher R, Tomita K. Does spinal surgery improve quality of life for those with extra-dural (spinal) osseus metastases? An international mutlicenter prospective observational study. *J Neurosurg Spine* 2008; **8**: 271–278.

Study design

* Multi-institutional, randomized trial

Class of evidence	I
Randomization	Surgery plus radiotherapy versus radiotherapy alone
Number of patients	101 randomized
Follow-up	Period of time not specified, but monthly assessment of all patients
	Primary outcomes: Ability to walk
	Secondary outcomes: Urinary continence, muscle strength and functional status, need for steroids and opiates, survival time
Number of centres	7
Stratification	Tumour type Spinal stability Ambulatory status Institution

* MESCC was defined radiologically as displacement of the spinal cord by an epidural mass.

* Inclusion criteria: Age > 18 years; at least one neurological sign; tissue diagnosis of non-CNS tumour; prognosis > 3 months.

* Exclusion criteria: Paraplegia > 48 h; radiosensitive tumour (lymphomas, leukaemia, multiple myeloma, germ cell tumour); previous MESCC.

- Patients received treatment within 24 h of randomization.
- Radiation dose was 3.0 Gy × 10 fractions.
- Surgery was to decompress the spinal cord but no constraints were placed on technique or methods of fixation.
- Surgical patients received radiotherapy within 14 days of surgery.

Outcome measures

Primary endpoint

- Ambulatory status: 'ambulant' was defined as taking two steps with each foot unassisted (cane or walker allowed).

Secondary endpoints

- Urinary continence
- Functional status: Frankel functional scale score
- Muscle strength: ASIA motor score
- Steroid use: calculation of mean daily doses

Results

- The trial was stopped early as interim analysis suggested that surgical therapy was superior.

Outcome	Surgery + DXT	DXT alone	Statistical significance
Patients with ability to walk after treatment	84%	57%	$p = 0.001$
Patients recovering ability to walk	62%	19%	$p = 0.01$
Patients retaining ability to walk	94%	74%	$p = 0.02$
Median time patients able to walk after treatment	122 days	13 days	$p = 0.003$

- Patients in the surgery group also did significantly better in all secondary outcomes (continence, functional scores, muscle strength, and less steroid use).

Conclusions

Surgical decompression with radiotherapy is superior to radiotherapy alone in MESCC.

Critique

MESCC is a significant problem and approximately 30% of cancer patients will develop symptomatic MESCC (Sciubba and Gokaslan, 2006). Although this disorder does not alter life expectancy, resultant neurological deficit significantly affects quality of life. This study does appear to show a benefit for surgery, although no direct comparison of radiotherapy alone.

Several criticisms have been made regarding this study (Ibrahim *et al.*, 2008) Firstly, there may have been selection bias in this study as the inclusion criteria were quite narrow. Patients with a prognosis of less than 3 months or who had been paraplegic for more than 48 h were excluded. Secondly, recruitment rates to the study were also low (approximately 1 patient per year over 10 years). Thirdly, the definition of 'ambulant' as '2 steps with each foot' is highly questionable.

Early studies looking at the role of laminectomy in MESCC had suggested that surgery may be associated with a poor outcome (Findlay, 1984). Radiotherapy alone has, therefore, become an accepted treatment regime for MESCC. However, methods of spinal fixation have significantly improved over recent years and it is now possible to undertake decompressive surgery in cases that were previously not deemed to be surgical candidates. This study by Patchell and colleagues has been highly significant in re-establishing the role of surgery in MESCC. Further studies are already beginning to follow to look at this complex clinical problem. One particularly good multi-centre observational study suggests that surgical decompression for MESCC is associated with an improved quality of life (Ibrahim *et al.*, 2008).

Findlay GF. Adverse effects of the management of malignant spinal cord compression. *J Neurol Neurosurg Psychiatry* 1984; **47**: 761–768.

Ibrahim A, Crockard A, Antonietti P, Boriani S, Bunger C, Gasbarrini A, Grejes A, Harms J, Kawahara N, Mazel C, Melcher R, Tomita K. Does spinal surgery improve quality of life for those with extradural (spinal) osseus metastases? An international mutlicenter prospective observational study. *J Neurosurg Spine* 2008; **8**: 271–278.

Sciubba DM, Gokaslan ZL. Diagnosis and management of metastatic spine disease. *Surgical Oncology* 2006; **15**: 141–151.

4.5 **Surgery for lumbar disc herniation**

There are three landmark trials that address the issue of surgical intervention for lumbar disc herniation. The first trial influenced practice for over 30 years (Weber, 1983). This was a single-centre study that followed up a randomized cohort of patients in which there was equipoise regarding surgical intervention and an observational cohort of patients in which it was felt there was no equipoise. The study took place in the Ullevall Hospital, Oslo, Norway, over a 10-year period between in the 1970s and 1980s. The second study was the SPORT (Weinstein *et al.*, 2006). SPORT was conducted in the United States between 2000 and 2004 and examined surgery versus conservative management for lumbar disc prolapse. The third was carried out by the Leiden – The Hague Spine Intervention Prognostic Study Group (Peul *et al.*, 2007; Peul *et al.*, 2008). This study looked at early surgery versus prolonged conservative management in the management of sciatica due to lumbar disc herniation and was carried out in the Netherlands between 2002 and 2005.

Study references

Main studies

Norwegian study (Weber, 1983)

Weber H. Lumbar disc herniation. A controlled, prospective study with ten years of observation. *Spine* 1983; **8**: 131–140.

US study: SPORT (Weinstein *et al.*, 2006)

Weinstein JN, Tosteson TD, Lurie JD, Tosteson ANA, Hnascom B, Skinner JS, Abdu WA, Hilibrand AS, Boden SD, Deyo RA. Surgical vs nonoperative treatment of lumbar disk herniation: the spine patient outcomes research trial (SPORT): a randomised trial. *JAMA* 2006; **296**: 2441–2450.

Netherlands study (Peul *et al.*, 2007)

Peul WC, van den Hout WB, Brand R, Thomeer RTWM, Koes BW, for the Leiden – The Hague Spine Intervention Prognostic Study Group. Prolonged conservative care versus early surgery in patients with sciatica caused by lumbar disc herniation: two year results of a randomised controlled trial. *BMJ* 2008; **336**: 1355–1358.

Peul WC, van Houwelingen HC, van den Hout WB, Brand R, Eekof JA,Tans JT, Thomeer RTWM, Koes BW for the Leiden – The Hague Spine Intervention Prognostic Study Group. Surgery versus prolonged conservative treatment for sciatica. *N Engl J Med* 2007; **356**: 2245–2256.

Related references

Fairbank J. Prolapsed intervertebral disc. *BMJ* 2008; **336**: 1317–1318.

Gibson JN, Waddell G. Surgical interventions for lumbar disc prolapse: updated Cochrane Review. *Spine* 2007; **32**: 1735–1747.

Gibson J, Grant I, Waddell G. The Cochrane review of surgery for lumbar disc prolapse and degenerative lumbar spondylosis. *Spine* 1999; **24**: 1820–1832.

Van den Hout WB, Peul WC, Koes BVW, Brand R, Klevit J, Thomeer RTWM for the Leiden – The Hague Spine Intervention Prognostic Study Group. Prolonged conservative care versus early surgery in patients with sciatica from lumbar disc herniation: cost utility analysis alongside a randomised controlled trial. *BMJ* 2008; **336**: 1351–1354.

Weinstein JN, Tosteson TD, Lurie JD, Tosteson ANA, Blood E, Hanscom B, Herkwoitz H, Cammisa F, Albert T, Boden SD, Hilibrand A, Goldberg H, Berven S, An H for the SPORT Investigators. Surgical versus nonsurgical therapy for lumbar spinal stenosis. *N Engl J Med* 2008; **358**: 794–810.

Weinstein JN, Lurie JD, Tosteson TD, Hanscom B, Tosteson ANA, Blood EA, Birkmeyer NJO, Hilibrand AS, Herkowitz H, Cammisa FP, Todd JA, Emery SE, Lenke LG, Abdu WA, Longley M, Errico TJ, Hu SS. Surgery versus nonsurgical treatment for lumbar degenerative spondylolisthesis. *New Engl J Med* 2007; **356**: 2257–2270.

Study designs

◆ All three studies involved randomization, but only the US and Netherlands studies were PRCT.

	Norwegian study	US study (SPORT)	Netherlands study
Class of evidence	III	II	II
Randomization	Surgery versus conservative management	Surgery versus conservative management	Early surgery versus conservative management
Number of patients	126	501	283
Follow-up	1, 4, and 10 years	2 years	2 years
	Primary outcomes: Neurological function and pain relief	Primary outcomes: Pain Physical function	Primary outcomes: Disability Relief of sciatica Perceived recovery
	Secondary outcomes: Functional status Quality of life	Secondary outcomes: Sciatica severity Patient satisfaction and self-reported improvement Employment status	Secondary outcomes: Quality of life Functional-economic status Back pain
Number of centres	1	13	9
Stratification	None	None	None

Inclusion and exclusion criteria

	Norwegian study	US study (SPORT)	Netherlands study
Inclusion criteria	Adult patients; sciatica (L5 and/or S1 root lesion)	Age ≥18, ≥6 weeks radicular pain and signs of nerve root irritation (or neurological deficit); radiological evidence of lumbar disc herniation (mostly MRI confirmation)	Age 18–65, radiculopathy of 6–12 weeks' duration; radiologically confirmed disc herniation at a level consistent with radiculopathy
Exclusion criteria	Spondylolisthesis; previous back surgery	Previous back surgery; CES; other serious back pathology; patients not wishing to contemplate surgery	Cauda equina syndrome or severe paresis; history of spinal surgery; spinal stenosis; severe co-morbidities

- In the Norwegian study, uncertainty regarding the indication for surgery triggered randomization.
- Surgery was standard open discectomy in all three studies.
- Surgery was performed within 2 weeks of randomization in the Netherlands study and was therefore early surgery.
- Analysis on an intention-to-treat basis for the US and Netherlands studies.

Outcome measures

	Norwegian study	US study (SPORT)	Netherlands study
Primary endpoints	Clinical evaluation: outcomes categorized as good, fair, poor, or bad	Pain measured using the Medical Outcomes Study 26-Item Short Form Survey (SF-36) which scores 0–100 with reducing severity Physical function also measured with the SF-36 and also the Oswestry Disability Index (ODI) which scores 0–100 with increasing severity	Disability: Roland questionnaire Leg pain: visual analogue scale Perceived recovery: Likert self-rating scale
Secondary endpoints	Quality of life: patient questionnaire	Sciatica severity: Sciatica Botherness Index (SBI) which scores 0–24 with increasing severity Patient satisfaction and reported improvement: percentage scale	Quality of life: QOL scales Functional-economic status (FES): observational scores Back pain: visual analogue scale

- In the Norwegian study the categorization of outcomes into four groups (good, fair, poor, bad) was based on an appraisal by the examining doctors at follow-up.

Results

Norwegian study

1 year outcomes	Conservative Management	Surgery	Statistical significance
Good	36%	65%	
Fair	42%	27%	$p = 0.0015$
Poor	20%	8%	
Bad	2%	0%	

- There was a statistically significant benefit of surgery at 1 year ($p = 0.0015$).
- Twenty-six percent of patients in the conservatively managed group were operated on during the first year. The results of surgery were statistically better whether or not these 26% of patients were included in the analysis.
- Beyond 4 years, although there was a trend towards benefit, the difference was not statistically significant.

US study (SPORT)

◆ Ninety-four percent follow-up at 1 year, but follow-up at 2 years was <80%.

Outcomes (12 months)	Surgery	Conservative management	Statistical significance
Pain (SF-36)	39.7	36.9	None
Physical function(SF-36)	36.4	35.2	None
ODI	−30.6	−27.4	None

◆ There was a statistically significant improvement of Sciatica Botherness Index (SBI) in the surgery group at 1 year compared to the conservatively managed group ($p = 0.003$).
◆ Self-rated progress favoured surgery ($p = 0.4$).
◆ There was significant cross-over between groups with: 40% of the surgical group; 45% of the conservatively managed group.
◆ An as-treated analysis indicated a benefit of surgery.

Netherlands study

◆ Follow-up was 99% at 1 year and 77% at 2 years.

	Surgery	Conservative management
Median time to recovery	4.0 weeks (95% CI, 3.7 to 4.3)	12.11 weeks (95% CI, 9.5 to 14.8)

◆ Early surgery produced a 17.7% better relief of leg pain compared to conservative treatment at 8 weeks.
◆ Inverse Kaplan–Meier curves were used to estimate the cumulative incidence of recovery: the hazard ratio was 1.97% in favour of early surgery (95% CI, 1.72 to 2.22).
◆ The short-term benefit of early surgery ceased to be statistically significant by 6 months.

Conclusions

Norwegian study

Surgical treatment was better than conservative management at 1-year follow-up, but this difference became less pronounced over a 10-year period.

US study (SPORT)

Patients received benefit from both surgery and conservative management but no conclusions regarding the superiority of either can be made on an intention-to-treat analysis.

Netherlands study

Early surgery for sciatica due to lumbar disc prolapse leads to faster recovery and relief of leg pain. However, there are no long-term benefits.

Critique

The natural history of sciatica due to lumbar disc herniation is such that the majority of patients will improve significantly within 8 weeks. Surgery is generally reserved for those patients who do not experience improvement within this time period. The Norwegian study by Weber appeared to demonstrate a benefit of surgery 1 year following surgery. Although this benefit was not seen at 4-year follow-up, this study influenced practice over the next two decades. This study would perhaps be criticized today for the methodology by which outcomes were assessed, which, on the whole, appears to be largely subjective assessments.

The US study (SPORT trial) did not show any differences between surgery and conservative management in the intention-to-treat analysis. However, this study is hampered by a number of weaknesses including the large number of cross-overs between treatment groups. Nonetheless, supporters of the trial argue that this reflects the reality of spinal practice and is the only way in which a trial for this condition can be carried out. The same arguments are made to support the use of an as-treated analysis. However, this methodology does not allow the exclusion of the placebo effect and the possibility of false-positive outcomes. Fairbank has made the point that the fact that 44% of the conservative arm switched to surgery reflects the impact of this condition on the patient (Fairbank, 2008).

The Netherlands study by Peul *et al.* differs from previous studies in that it evaluated the role of early surgery (within 2 weeks of randomization). In addition, Peul *et al.* specifically looked at the speed of recovery between conservative and surgical groups. Their study shows that although surgery results in faster recovery compared to conservative management, there is no overall difference in the longer-term outcomes. The findings of this study are upheld in an updated Cochrane review of published studies on lumbar disc surgery, which concluded that, for carefully selected patients with sciatica due to lumbar disc herniation, surgery provides a faster relief from the acute attack than conservative management (Gibson and Waddell, 2007).

The lack of any long-term benefit following surgery means that the risks of surgery need to be balanced against the risks of conservative management. Surgical risks include a 1% risk of neurological damage. However, the risks of conservative management have not been quantified in sciatica and may include further neurological deterioration and the development of cauda equina syndrome (Fairbank, 2008). There are, therefore, insufficient data to justify surgical intervention in lumbar disc herniation on the balancing of risks. However, there may be a rationale for early surgical intervention based on a cost–benefit analysis. The cost of surgical intervention can be weighed against the cost of lost productivity for the longer period of recovery in patients managed conservatively. The authors of the Netherlands study went on to examine this cost–benefit analysis and found that there appears to be a strong economic argument supporting continued surgery for lumbar disc herniations producing sciatica (van den Hout *et al.*, 2008).

In summary, sciatica due to lumbar disc herniation is a common problem. However, there is still controversy regarding the natural history of this disorder. The trials reviewed here are landmarks in the field of neurosurgery as they have provided valuable information regarding the natural history of this disorder and its treatment.

Fairbank J. Prolapsed intervertebral disc. *BMJ* 2008; **336**: 1317–1318.

Gibson JNA, Waddell G. Surgical interventions for lumbar disc prolapse: Updated Cochrane Review. *Spine* 2007; **32**: 1735–1747.

Van den Hout WB, Peul WC, Koes BVW, Brand R, Klevit J, Thomeer RTWM for the Leiden – The Hague Spine Intervention Prognostic Study Group. Prolonged conservative care versus early surgery in patients with sciatica from lumbar disc herniation: cost utility analysis alongside a randomised controlled trial. *BMJ* 2008; **336**: 1351–1354.

4.6 **Microscopic sequestrectomy for lumbar disc herniation**

Details of study

This prospective randomized study aimed to evaluate whether there was any difference in outcomes in patients undergoing standard microdiscectomy or microscopic sequestration of disc fragments. The study was carried out in a single centre in Heidelberg in Germany.

Study references

Main study

Barth M, Diepers M, Weiss C, Thome C . Two-year outcome after lumbar microdiscectomy versus microscopic sequestrectomy: part1: evaluation of clinical outcome. *Spine* 2008; **33**: 265–272.

Related references

Barth M, Diepers M, Weiss C, Thome C. Two-year outcome after lumbar microdiscectomy versus microscopic sequestrectomy: part 2: radiographic evaluation and correlation with clinical outcome. *Spine* 2008; **33**: 273–279.

Caspar W. A new surgical procedure for lumbar disc herniation causing less tissue damage through a microsurgical approach. *Adv Neurosurg* 1977; **4**: 74–77.

Thome C, Barth M, Schard *et al*. Outcome after lumbar sequestrectomy compared with microdiscectomy: a prospective randomised study. *J Neurosurg Spine* 2005; **2**: 271–278.

Williams RW. Microlumbar discectomy: a conservative surgical approach to the virgin herniated lumbar disc. *Spine* 1978; **3**: 175–182.

Yasargil MG. Microsurgical operation of herniated disc. *Adv Neurosurg* 1977; **4**: 81–82.

Study design

- Single-centre PRCT.

Class of evidence	II
Randomization	Standard microdiscectomy versus sequestrectomy
Number of patients	84
Follow-up	2 years
	Primary outcomes: Neurological status Clinical symptoms Quality of life
	Secondary outcomes: Reherniation rates Functional and economic status
Number of centres	1

- Inclusion criteria: Age 18–60 years; no previous lumbar surgery; MRI confirmation of lumbar disc prolapse; no concomitant spinal disease.
- Standard discectomy involved removal of herniated disc matter and clearance of the disc space.
- Sequestrectomy involved removal of loose disc material and the disc space was not entered.

Outcome measures

Primary endpoints

- Neurological status was established by clinical neurological examination.
- Quality of life was assessed using the SF-36 questionnaire.

Secondary endpoints

- Functional and economic status were assessed using Prolo scores from questionnaires.

Results

- Follow-up was 93% at 2 years.
- There was no statistical difference in the reherniation rates: 12.5% sequestrectomy; 10% discectomy.
- There was no difference in neurological status or clinical symptomatology between the two groups.
- An analysis of overall outcome suggested that there was a statistically significant better overall outcome with sequestrectomy at 2 years ($p = 0.004$) and a significantly greater improvement of overall outcome over time with sequestrectomy ($p = 0.029$)
- There appeared to be a statistically significant benefit of surgery in terms of parameters assessed by questionnaires including quality of life.

Conclusions

Sequestrectomy may be advantageous compared to standard microdiscectomy and reherniation rates are similar with both techniques.

Critique

In their earlier publication, the same authors had shown that there was no difference in outcome between the two techniques at 6-month follow-up (Thome *et al.*, 2005). This study extends these findings from that study to 2-year follow-up. However, the study includes two operating surgeons only at a single institution and is hindered by problems of blinding.

The authors of the study attack what they refer to as 'discectomy dogma' which holds that unless the disc space is cleared there remains a risk of reherniation, subsequent nerve root compression, and clinical deterioration. In order support their view that there is no scientific basis for this, the authors also carried out a radiological follow-up study by way of MRI on their cohort of patients (Barth *et al.*, 2008). They report that sequestrectomy was associated with less post-operative disc degeneration and end-plate changes.

Although this trial is a single-centre, unblinded study, it provokes substantial questions regarding the accepted rationale behind standard microdiscectomy and certainly paves the way for larger multi-centre trials.

Barth M, Diepers M, Weiss C, Thome C. Two-year outcome after lumbar microdiscectomy versus microscopic sequestrectomy: part 2: radiographic evaluation and correlation with clinical outcome. *Spine* 2008; **33**: 273–279.

Thome C, Barth M, Schard *et al.* Outcome after lumbar sequestrectomy compared with microdiscectomy: a prospective randomised study. *J Neurosurg Spine* 2005; **2**: 271–278.

4.7 Surgery for cauda equina syndrome

Details of studies

There is no prospective randomized trial evaluating the timing of surgery for CES. However, case series reported in the literature have strongly supported the view that CES is a diagnostic and surgical emergency and that early surgery results in a better outcome than delayed surgery (O'Laoire *et al.*, 1981; Hellström *et al.*, 1986; Dinning and Schaefer, 1993; Shapiro, 1993; Kennedy *et al.*, 1999; Chang *et al.*, 2000; Shapiro, 2000). In this section, we have summarized the findings from these case series regarding the timing of surgery and sphincter function. Two meta-analyses of published case series have been carried out, one by Ahn *et al.* and one by Todd (Ahn *et al.*, 2000; Todd, 2005; Jerwood and Todd, 2006). The meta-analysis carried out by Todd included all the case series listed here.

Study references

Main studies

Case series

Chang HS, Nakaagawa H, Mizuno J. Lumbar herniated disc presenting with cauda equine syndrome. Long-term follow-up of four cases. *Surg Neurol* 2000; **53**: 100–105.

Dinning TAR, Schaefer HR. Discogenic compression of the cauda equina: a surgical emergency. *Aust NZ J Surg* 1993; **63**: 927–934.

Hellström P, Kortelainen P, Kontturi M. Late urodynamic findings after surgery for cauda equine syndrome caused by a prolapsed lumbar intervertebral disk. *J Urol* 1986; **135**: 308–312.

Kennedy JG, Soffe KE, McGrath A, Stephens MM, Walsh MG, McManus F. Predictors of outcome in cauda equina syndrome. *Eur J Spine* 1999; **8**: 317–322.

O'Laoire SA, Crockard HA, Thomas DG. Prognosis for sphinctor recovery after operation for operaton for cauda equina compression owing to lumbar disc prolapse. *BMJ* 1981; **282**: 1852–1854.

Shapiro S. Cauda equina syndrome secondary to lumbar disc herniation. *Neurosurgery* 1993; **32**: 743–747.

Shapiro S. Medical realities of cauda equina syndrome secondary to lumbar disc herniation. *Spine* 2000; **25**: 348–351.

Meta-analyses

Ahn UM, Ahn NU, Buchowski MS, Garrett ES, Sieber AN, Kostuik JP. Cauda equina syndrome secondary to lumbar disc herniation. A meta-analysis of surgical outcomes. *Spine* 2000; **25**: 1515–1522.

Todd NV. Cauda equina syndrome: the timing of surgery probably does influence outcome. *B J Neurosurg* 2005; **19**: 301–306.

Jerwood D, Todd NV. Reanalysis of the timing of cauda equina surgery. *Br J Neurosurg* 2006; **20**: 178–179.

Related references

Findlay G. Meta-analysis and the timing of cauda equina surgery. *B J Neurosurg* 2008; **22**: 137–138.

Gleave JR, MacFarlane R. Cauda equina syndrome: what is the relationship between timing of surgery and outcome. *B J Neurosurg* 2002; **16**: 325–328.

McFarlane R. Meta-analysis and the timing of cauda equina surgery. *B J Neurosurg* 2007; **21**: 635.

Case series

Study designs

◆ All retrospective analysis of case series.

Results

Series	Number of patients	Findings	Conclusion
O'Laoire et al. (1981)	29	◆ No correlation between the length of the history and the outcome from surgery ◆ Preservation of sphincter function was better than expected	Emergency operation is mandatory for CES
Hellström et al. (1986)	17	◆ 66% of patients operated on within 48 h recovered sphincter function ◆ 50% of patients operated on after 48 h recovered sphincter function	Bladder dysfunction can occur in CES without symptoms and emergency surgery can reduce later bladder dysfunction
Dinning and Schaefer (1993)	39	◆ 88% operated on within 24 h showed recovery of sphincter dysfunction ◆ Only 20% of patients operated on after 24 h showed recovery of sphincter dysfunction	CES is a surgical emergency with bladder dysfunction being the most important indication for surgery
Shapiro (1993)	14	◆ 100% of patients operated on within 48 h regained continence and unassisted ambulation ◆ 100% of patients with persistent incontinence underwent surgery after >48 h	CES is a surgical emergency and every effort should be made to operate within 24 to 48 h of onset
Kennedy et al. (1999)	19	◆ Mean time to decompression with a satisfactory outcome was 14 h ◆ Mean time to decompression with a poor outcome was 30 h ◆ Delayed surgery was significantly associated with poor outcome ($p = 0.023$)	Early diagnosis and early decompression are associated with a favourable outcome
Chang et al. (2000)	4	◆ Although sphincter function was poor in the early post-operative period this improved over the long term	Long-term sphincter function may be better than the short-term results of surgery
Shapiro (2000)	44	◆ Delayed surgery (>48 h) is associated with significant sphincter dysfunction ($p = 0.008$)	CES is a diagnostic and surgical emergency

Meta-analyses

Study designs

Ahn *et al.* (2000)

- Logistic regression analysis was carried out to determine correlation between timing of surgery and clinical outcomes.
- The authors compartmentalized timing of surgery into five groups: <24 h; 24–48 h; 2–10 days; 11 days to 1 month; >1 month.

Todd (2005)

- Todd looked at patients in the literature who had been operated on within 24 h or 48 h from onset of CES and developed two null hypotheses:

  1 There is no benefit to early decompression within 24 h.

  2 There is no benefit to early decompression within 48 h.

- Todd, therefore, analysed the literature with only one input variable, being the timing of surgery.
- The only output variable analysed was recovery of sphincter function defined as 'socially normal bladder function'.
- Statistical significance of odds ratios were calculated for the benefits of decompression on sphincter function in early versus late surgery.

Results

Analysis	Findings	Conclusions
Ahn *et al.* (2000)	There was no significant benefit of surgery within 24 h or after 48 h There was a significant beneficial effect of surgery between 24 and 48 h	There is a benefit to surgery performed within 48 h
Todd (2005)	The probability of benefit from surgery within 24 h is $p = 0.03$ The probability of benefit from surgery within 48 h is $p = 0.005$	The timing of surgery following CES probably influence outcome

Critique

The first description of neurological compromise from a ruptured lumbar intervertebral disc was published in 1934 (Mixter and Barr, 1934). In 1959, Shephard published a review of CES cases presenting to Maida Vale Hospital, London, and concluded that early surgery was necessary to minimize permanent neurological damage (Shephard, 1959). O'Laoire *et al.* followed on from Shepard in their report of a series of patients with CES presenting to the National Hospitals for Nervous Diseases at Queen Square and Maida Vale, and University College London, between 1960 and 1980 (O'Laoire *et al.*, 1981).

O'Laoire *et al.* expressed their opinion regarding the management of this condition in no uncertain terms:

> *The urgency of the diagnosis and treatment may be compared to that for extradural haematoma in head injury.*

O'Laoire *et al.* (1981)

This is representative of the prevailing view regarding the timing of surgery for CES. The summary of conclusions from the case series included here reflects this view also. The meta-analysis carried out by Ahn *et al.* has received strong criticism for methodology and design. Indeed, it has been maintained that the logistic regression analysis performed by Ahn *et al.* is not a meta-analysis at all as it includes widely diverse patient populations with incomparable input and output variables (Kohles *et al.*, 2004; Todd, 2005). The meta-analysis performed by Todd is certainly more rigorous in the application of the rules of meta-analysis and they demonstrated a statistically significant disproval of both their null hypotheses. Furthermore, in a re-analysis of Todd's meta-analysis, Jerwood and Todd concluded that there is 'overwhelming statistical evidence' for the benefit of surgery to be performed as soon as is practically possible (Jerwood and Todd, 2006). McFarlane has criticized the conclusions drawn from the meta-analysis of on several grounds (McFarlane, 2007). Firstly, McFarlane argues that it does not make physiological sense that patients with a complete CES should show signs of recovery up to 24 h after compression: larger peripheral nerves suffer irreversible injury after only a few hours. Secondly, McFarlane expresses the view that emergency surgery can be associated with increased morbidity as it may be carried out in suboptimal conditions out of hours. Furthermore, Gleave and McFarlane have indicated that in many of the reported series catheter placement may have been erroneously equated with loss of sphincter function (Gleave and McFarlane, 2002). Findlay has also objected that re-analysis by Jerwood and Todd places too much emphasis on the later series from Shapiro *et al.* which may have included smaller discs than are typical of CES (Findlay, 2008). Findlay's critique concluded that whilst the benefit of surgery for CES within 24 h remains unanswered it appears clear that an evolving case of CES will likely prevent further neurological deterioration. The answers to these questions have implications for resource management, consent, and medicolegal causality of neurological disability. It is possible that further studies will have to include some form of dynamic bladder function measurements in order to determine more accurately the extent of the CES perioperatively.

Kohles SS, Kohles DA, Kar AP, Erlich VM, Polissar NL. Time-dependent surgical outcomes following cauda equina syndrome diagnosis: comments on a meta-analysis. *Spine* 2004; **29**: 1281–1287.

Mixter JM, Barr JS. Ruputre of the intervertebral disc with involvement of the spinal canal. *N Eng J Med* 1934; **211**: 210–215.

Shephard RH. Diagnosis and prognosis of cauda equine syndrome produced by protrusion of lumbar disc. *BMJ* 1959; **ii**: 1434–1439.

4.8 **Surgery for lumbar stenosis**

Details of study

As part of the SPORT trial carried out in the United States, the investigators assessed the role of decompressive laminectomy versus conservative management in the treatment of lumbar stenosis.

Study references

Main study

Weinstein JN, Tosteson TD, Lurie JD, Tosteson ANA, Blood E, Hanscom B, Herkwoitz H, Cammisa F, Albert T, Boden SD, Hilibrand A, Goldberg H, Berven S, An H for the SPORT Investigators. Surgical versus nonsurgical therapy for lumbar spinal stenosis. *N Engl J Med* 2008; **358**: 794–810.

Related reference

Weinstein JN, Lurie JD, Tosteson TD, Hanscom B, Tosteson ANA, Blood EA, Birkmeyer NJO, Hilibrand AS, Herkowitz H, Cammisa FP, Todd JA, Emery SE, Lenke LG, Abdu WA, Longley M, Errico TJ, Hu SS. Surgery versus nonsurgical treatment for lumbar degenerative spondylolisthesis. *New Engl J Med* 2007; **356**: 2257–2270.

Study design

- RCT plus concomitant observational cohort

Class of evidence	II
Randomization	Decompressive laminectomy versus conservative care
Number of patients	289
Follow-up	2 years
	Primary outcomes: Bodily pain Physical function
	Secondary outcomes: Patient reported improvement
Number of centres	13
Stratification	None

- There was also a concurrent observational cohort of 365 patients who refused randomization.
- Inclusion criteria: ≥12 weeks neurogenic claudication and radiological evidence of lumbar stenosis.
- Exclusion criteria: Lumbar spondylolisthesis; lumbar instability (defined radiologically on lateral lumbar films).

Outcome measures

Primary endpoints

- Pain measured using the Medical Outcomes Study 26-Item Short Form Survey (SF-36) which scores 0–100 with reducing severity
- Physical function also measured with the SF-36 and also the Oswestry Disability Index (ODI) which scores 0–100 with increasing severity
- Outcomes were measured as changes from baseline scores

Secondary endpoint

- Patient-reported improvement

Results

- Randomized cohort: 85% follow-up at 1 year; 76% follow-up at 2 years.
- Observational cohort: 92% follow-up at 1 year; 88% follow-up at 2 years.
- Cross-over: 42% of those randomized to conservative management had undergone surgery at 1 year compared to 63% of those randomized to surgery.

Primary outcomes of randomized cohort at 1 and 2 years (intention-to-treat analysis):

Primary outcomes		Surgery	Conservative Care	Statistical significance
Bodily pain (Change in SF-36)	1 year	23	18	None
	2 years	23	16	Yes ($p < 0.05$?)
Physical function (Change in SF-36)	1 year	18	16	None
	2 years	17	17	None
Disability (Change in ODI)	1 year	−15	−13	None
	2 years	−16	−13	None

- In an as-treated analysis there appeared to be a benefit of surgery on primary outcomes in both randomized and observational cohorts.

Conclusions

Surgery is better than conservative care in the management of lumbar stenosis.

Critique

Follow-up in the randomized cohort was <80% at 2 years and so there is doubt regarding the validity of the observed benefit of surgery on bodily pain at 2 years. At 1 year where there was >80% follow-up there were no differences in the primary outcomes in the intention-to-treat analysis. Differences reported an as-treated analysis that combined both randomized and observational cohorts. There were difficulties with high cross-over rates in the randomized cohort and it appeared that patients crossing over to surgery had different demographics.

The SPORT trial also included a similarly designed study that looked at a randomized cohort and a non-randomized cohort of patients undergoing surgery or non-operative care for lumbar spine degenerative spondylolisthesis (Weinstein *et al.*, 2007). This study also had the same problems due to the high rates of cross-over between treatment groups and only an as-treated analysis showed a favourable effect of surgery.

The SPORT studies are important because they show the inherent difficulties in carrying out randomized controlled trials in spinal patients. However, the studies may reflect the realities of spinal practice and any criticism of their inherent weakness needs to be weighed with this in mind.

Weinstein JN, Lurie JD, Tosteson TD, Hanscom B, Tosteson ANA, Blood EA, Birkmeyer NJO, Hillibrand AS, Herkowitz H, Cammisa FP, Albert TJ, Emery SE, Lenke LG, Abdu WA, Longley M, Errico TJ, Hu SS. Surgical versus nonsurgical treatment for lumbar degenerative spondylolisthesis. *New Engl J Med* 2007; **356**: 2257–2270.

4.9 **Spinal stabilization for chronic back pain**

Details of study

The MRC spine stabilization trial was carried out in response to the NHS standing group on health technology in 1994 concluding that there was weak evidence for surgery in chronic low back pain. The trial was carried out in 15 secondary care orthopaedic and rehabilitation centres across the United Kingdom.

Study references

Main study

Fairbank J, Frost H, Wilson-MacDonald J, Yu LM, Barker K, Collins R and for the Spine Stabilisation Trial Group. Randomised controlled trial to compare surgical stabilisation of the lumbar spine with an intensive rehabilitation programme for patients with chronic low back pain: the MRC spine stabilisation trial. *BMJ* 2005; **330**: 1233–1240.

Related reference

Fritzell P, Hagg O, Wessburg P, Nordwall A, Group SLSS. Chronic back pain and fusion: a comparison of three surgical techniques: a prospective randomised controlled trial from the Swedish Lumbar Spine Study Group. *Spine* 2002; **27**: 1131–1141.

Study design

* PRCT

Class of evidence	I
Randomization	Lumbar spine fusion versus intensive rehabilitation
Number of patients	349
Follow-up	2 years
	Primary outcomes: Back pain Mobility
	Secondary outcomes: General health assessment Psychological assessment Complications
Number of centres	15

* Inclusion criteria: Clinician and patient uncertainty regarding which treatment option is best; ≥12 months of chronic lower back pain; age 18–55 years.

* Exclusion criteria: Previous stabilization surgery; significant co-morbidities; pregnancy; psychiatric disease.

* Choice of surgical method of stabilization was left to the discretion of the operating surgeon.

- Rehabilitation programmes were outpatient-based with similar intensity regimes employed between study centres.
- Analysis was on an intention-to-treat basis.

Outcome measures

Primary endpoints

- Back pain: ODI; 0 = no disability, 100 = severe disability
- Mobility: Shuttle-walking test (SWT) which measures maximal walking distance in metres

Secondary endpoints

- General health assessment: the Medical Outcomes Study 26-Item Short Form Survey (SF-36)
- Psychological assessment: distress and risk assessment method (modified Zung depression index and sensory perception questionnaire)

Results

- Eighty-one percent follow-up at 2 years.
- Cross-over: 28% of patients randomized to rehabilitation had undergone surgery by 2 years; 7% of patients randomized to surgery had rehabilitation instead of surgery.
- There was small but statistically significant effect of surgery in improving ODI scores: -4.1 ($p = 0.045$).
- There was no difference in any of the other outcome measures.

Conclusions

There is no clear evidence for the benefit of surgery over rehabilitation in the treatment of chronic low back pain patients.

Critique

Although there were cross-overs and the follow-up was just over the 80% level this study represents one of the best designed and carried-out spinal studies. Problems included slow recruitment due to eligibility on uncertainty of outcome principle. It is possible, therefore, that 'certainty' may have excluded the best surgical candidates. Nonetheless this is an important study and the authors point out that the benefit of surgery is small compared to the cost and risks of surgery. The requirement for comprehensive rehabilitation services is emphasized by their results.

4.10 Surgery for cervical spondylotic myelopathy

Details of study

The largest trial comparing surgery with conservative measures for the treatment of cervical spondylotic myelopathy was a 3-year prospective randomized study carried out between 1993 and 2000 in the Czech Republic.

Study references

Main study

Kadanka Z, Mares M, Bednarik J, Smrcka V, Krbec M, Stejskal L, Chaloupka R, Surelova D, Novotny O, Urbanek I, Dusek L. Approaches to spondylotic cervical myelopathy: conservative versus surgical results in a 3-year follow-up study. *Spine* 2002; **27**: 2205–2211.

Related references

Kadanka Z, Bednarik J, Vohanka S, Vlach O, Stejskal L, Chaloupka R, Filipovicova D, Surelova D, Adamova B, Novotny O, Nemex M, Smrcka V, Urbanek I. Conservative treatment versus surgery in spondylotic cervical myelopathy: a prospective randomized study. *Eur Spine J* 2000; **9**: 538–544.

Kadanka Z, Mares M, Bednarik J, Smrcka V, Krbec M, Chaloupka R, Dusek L. Predictive factors for spondylotic cervical myelopathy treated conservatively or surgically. *Eur J Neurol* 2005; **12**: 55–63.

Study design

Class of evidence	II
Randomization	Surgery versus conservative management
Number of patients	68
Follow-up	3 years
	Primary endpoint: Clinical improvement
Number of centres	1
Stratification	Age

- Inclusion Criteria: Clinical cervical cord dysfunction; radiological evidence of cord compression on MRI; age <75 years; a modified Japanese Orthopaedic Association (mJOA) score of ≥12.
- Exclusion criteria: Contraindications to surgery; pervious surgery; other significant neurological disease.
- The majority of patients undergoing surgery underwent anterior decompression.
- Analysis was on an intention-to-treat basis.

Outcomes assessment

Primary endpoints

- Cervical cord function was graded clinically using the mJOA, which gives a total score out of 18.

- Mobility was assessed using a timed 10-m walk.
- Video-monitoring and patient self-evaluation of daily activities were also employed.

Results

- No significant difference was detected in the mJOA scores over the 3-year period.
- There was a small but significant improvement in the 10-m walk favouring those treated conservatively.
- There were no significant differences found between the two groups in evaluation of daily activities.

Conclusion

The authors concluded that, on average, their study did not show that surgery is superior to conservative therapy for the treatment of cervical spondylotic myelopathy.

Critique

One of the greatest weaknesses of this study was the small sample size. There is a possibility of a Type 2 error as power calculations indicate that a 42% difference in mJOA would need to be seen in order to detect a significant difference with the number of patients included in this study (Matz et al., 2009). Nonetheless, the results of this study are in keeping with a similar study that also included electrophysiological data (Bednarik et al., 1999).

In a further analysis of their data, the authors found that older patients appeared to do better with conservative treatment (Kadanka et al., 2005).

Bednarik J, Kadanka Z, Vohanka S, Stejskal L, Vlach O, Schroder R. The value of somatosensory- and motor-evoked potentials in predicting and monitoring the effect of therapy in spondylotic cervical myelopathy. Prospective randomized study. *Spine* 1999; **24**: 1593–1598.

Kadanka Z, Mares M, Bednarik J, Smrcka V, Krbec M, Chaloupka R, Dusek L. Predictive factors for spondylotic cervical myelopathy treated conservatively or surgically. *Eur J Neurol* 2005; **12**: 55–63.

Matz PG, Holly LT, Mummaneni PV, Anderson PA, Groff MW, Heary RF, Kaiser MG, Ryken TC, Choudhri TF, Vresilovic EJ, Resnick DK. Anterior cervical surgery for the treatment of cervical degenerative myelopathy. *J Neurosurg Spine* 2009; **11**: 170–173.

4.11 **Surgery for cervical radiculopathy**

Details of study

There is only one prospective randomized trial that has compared surgery with conservative management for cervical radiculopathy. This study was carried out in Lund, Sweden, and compared surgery, physiotherapy, and immobilization with a cervical collar.

Study references

Main reference

Persson LCG, Moritz U, Brandt L, Carlsson CA. Cervival radiculopathy: pain, muscle weakness and sensory loss in patients with cervical radiculopathy treated with surgery, physiotherahy or cervical collar. A prospective controlled study. *Eur Spine J* 1997; **6**: 256–266.

Related reference

Fouyas IP, Statham FX, Sandercock PAG. Cochrane review on the role of surgery in cervical spondylytic radiculomeyopathy. *Spine* 2002; **27**: 736–747.

Study design

- ◆ Single-centre PRT

Class of evidence	II
Randomization	Surgery versus physiotherapy versus immobilization with rigid cervical collar
Number of patients	81
Follow-up	16 months
	Primary endpoints: Relief of radicular pain Relief of sensory loss/paraesthesia Muscle strength
Number of centres	1
Stratification	None

- ◆ Inclusion criteria: Clinical and radiological evidence of cervical radiculopathy without spinal cord compression.
- ◆ Exclusion criteria: Cervical cord compression; whiplash; psychiatric co-morbidities.
- ◆ Surgery was primarily anterior cervical discectomy and fusion with a Cloward technique.
- ◆ Analysis was on an intention-to-treat basis.
- ◆ Follow-up was 98% at 16 months.

Outcome measures

Primary endpoints

- ◆ Pain was measured with a visual analogue scale: current pain and worst pain in the preceding week were scored.

- Sensory loss and paraesthesis were assessed by clinical examination by a physiotherapist.
- Muscle strength was measured using several dynamic devices.

Results

- At 3 months, patients undergoing surgery had statistically significantly less pain compared to those who received physiotherapy and those who underwent treatment in a rigid collar.

	Surgery	Physiotherapy	Rigid collar	Statistical significance
Reduction in Visual Analogue Score for pain at 3 months follow-up	29%	19%	4%	$p<0.05$

- At 1 year, there was no difference in the relief of pain between any of the groups.
- Although there was a significant relief of sensory loss/paraesthesia in the surgical group at 4 months, there was no difference between any of the three groups at 16 months follow-up.
- Muscle strength was slightly better in the surgery group at 4 months but there were no differences at 16 months.

Conclusion

Surgery results in a more rapid relief of radicular pain, sensory loss, and muscle weakness compared to conservative measures although the longer-term outcomes appear to be similar.

Critique

Previous prospective studies comparing pain relief of surgery versus conservative treatment suggested a benefit of surgery (De Palma and Subin, 1965). However, the study by Persson *et al.* was the first randomized study that evaluated surgery to conservative measures that included an assessment of motor and sensory function. The main criticisms of this trial are the non-blinding of physiotherapist assessor and the small sample size that could result in a Type 2 error (Fouyas *et al.*, 2002). However, the results of this study are in concordance with the results of previously published series and it remains the best level of evidence regarding surgery for cervical radiculopathy.

De Palma AF, Subin DK. Study of the cervical syndrome. *Clin Orthop* 1965; **38**: 135–141.

Fouyas IP, Statham FX, Sandercock PAG. Cochrane review on the role of surgery in cervical spondylytic radiculomeyopathy. *Spine* 2002; **27**: 736–747.

Chapter 5

Functional and epilepsy neurosurgery

AL Green, RD Johnson, A Astradsson,
RJ Stacey, TZ Aziz

5.0 **Introduction**

For this chapter, we have selected some landmark studies in the field of epilepsy and functional neurosurgery. These two subspecialty areas have become closer over recent years due to the wider use of stimulation procedures to control epilepsy, including vagal nerve stimulation (VNS).

The first epilepsy surgery study discussed is the trial by Wiebe *et al.* evaluating the efficacy of surgery in temporal lobe epilepsy refractory to medical management, which was published in the *New England Journal of Medicine* in 2001 (Wiebe *et al.*, 2001). This study was the first randomized controlled trial (RCT) assessing the efficacy of surgery for temporal lobe epilepsy. This trial has received widespread acclaim for confirming the efficacy of surgical intervention in epilepsy. Engel has pointed out that the results of this trial have laid open the question as to whether surgery should be considered earlier rather than as a last resort in medically refractory temporal lobe epilepsy (Engel, 2001). It is worth noting the circumstances in which it was possible to conduct this trial as surgical intervention is such a well-established method of treating temporal lobe epilepsy. The waiting list for temporal lobe surgery was 12 months and so this allowed Wiebe *et al.* to fast-track patients randomized to surgery to almost immediate pre-operative evaluation. This allowed for the ethical randomization of patients with a 12-month window to compare the two treatment arms. In the second section, we continue with the theme of epilepsy surgery and consider the two largest double-blind randomized trials evaluating VNS for the treatment of epilepsy (Ben-Menachem *et al.*, 1994; Handforth *et al.*, 1998).

The next sections of this chapter deal with functional neurosurgery by way of deep brain stimulation (DBS) and its indications. Functional neurosurgery encompasses brain lesioning and DBS in order to alter brain function. DBS was made possible by combining stereotactic methods with advances in neuromodulatory apparatus (neurostimulators) and in the better understanding of the functional anatomy of the deep nuclei of the brain. Stereotactic apparatus was introduced by Horsley and Clarke and further developed for surgical use by Spiegel and Wycis (Horsley and Clarke, 1908; Spiegel *et al.*, 1947). The advent of stereotactic methods has facilitated the development of two related fields of neurosurgery: functional neurosurgery and stereotactic radiosurgery.

DBS was first used clinically in the management of cancer pain and was then applied to a myriad of pain syndromes over the next 40 years. DBS for pain has predominantly been evaluated by case series rather than larger multi-centre controlled trials. However, a meta-analysis of DBS for pain relief concluded that it is effective in well-selected patients (Bittar *et al.*, 2005). Many of the developments in DBS for movement disorders have been the result of preclinical primate-based research and these in many ways are the real landmark studies in the history of this field of DBS. For example, the identification of the subthalamic nucleus (STN) as a target for DBS in the treatment of Parkinson's disease (PD) was the direct result of findings in primate models (Bergman *et al.*, 1990; Aziz *et al.*, 1991). However, as the aim of this volume is to highlight landmark clinical studies we have chosen to include three studies of DBS for movement disorders that we feel meet this criterion. We have included a clinical trial of neurostimulation versus sham stimulation of the globus pallidus internus (GPi) for dystonia (Kupsch *et al.*, 2006). Secondly, we have considered three studies evaluating STN DBS for PD. The first of these is a long-term follow-up study evaluating the efficacy of STN stimulation (Krack *et al.*, 2003). The second is a randomized trial comparing STN DBS to medical management. The third is the first randomized trial of best medical therapy versus STN DBS (Weaver *et al.*, 2009). We envisage that in future editions of this volume the findings of the UK 'PDSurg' trial will also be included.

Another area in which DBS is gaining an interested following is functional neurosurgery for psychiatric disorders. This area was formerly referred to as 'psychosurgery' and has, regrettably, a rather notorious history that has held back development in this field. It is worth, therefore, considering this history briefly here. It is likely that 'psychosurgery' may have an ancient pedigree with literature on trephination for psychosis dating back to 1500 BC (Mashour *et al.*, 2005). The first modern psychosurgical procedure was performed by Gottlieb Burckhardt when he carried out 'topectomy' (the removal of multiple foci of cerebral cortex) for psychosis in the late 19th century but (Burckhardt, 1891). However, it was in the first half of the 20th century that the Europeans Egas Moniz and Almeida Lima developed the prefrontal leucotomy for psychosis (Moniz, 1937). Although Moniz coined the term 'psychosurgery' and was awarded the Nobel Prize in 1949, the field took a downturn following the work of Walter Freeman who developed the transorbital frontal leucotomy with fellow American James Watts (Freeman, 1948). Although developed with the best of intentions, it is unfortunate that this procedure entered widespread, and often indiscriminate, use in the hands of non-surgically trained psychiatrists and physicians with such widespread complications that it was eventually rejected by most neurosurgeons, and indeed made illegal in some countries. This, combined with the introduction of an effective antipsychotic, chlorpromazine, into the pharmacopoeia, resulted in the effective death of 'psychosurgery'. There is, perhaps, some irony in the fact that the use of chlorpromazine as an antipsychotic stemmed from the observations of the French neurosurgeon Henri Laborit. Despite the decline of frontal lobectomy, other lesioning procedures have survived the test of time including cingulotomy for obsessive-compulsive disorder (OCD), which was made popular by Ballantyne (Ballantyne *et al.*, 1967). With the advent of DBS the field of functional neurosurgery is making inroads again into the realms of psychiatric disorders. We have included in this chapter the study by Mayberg *et al.* in Toronto that evaluates subgenual cingulated white matter as a target for DBS in treatment-resistant depression (Mayberg *et al.*, 2005). Although this is a pilot study, it represents a landmark in functional neurosurgery for extrapolating observations from functional imaging studies to develop a testable hypothesis regarding new efficacious targets for DBS in a major debilitating disorder.

Stereotactic radiosurgery was conceived by Lars Leksell of the Karolinska Institute in Stockholm (Leksell, 1951). Leksell combined stereotactic localization with radiation physics and together with Börge Larsson developed the Leksell gamma knife (Leksell, 1983). Stereotactic radiosurgery, therefore, allows the delivery of focal ablative lesions to a closed cranium and has been deployed successfully in the management of vascular malformations (AVMs), benign tumours (vestibular schwannomas and meningiomas), and pain syndromes (trigeminal neuralgia). Pollock, in a review of the clinical evidence for the efficacy of stereotactic radiosurgery, found that the majority of studies provided only Level III evidence (Pollock, 2006). This in part reflects the widespread establishment of this technique over the last 30 years. However, there are two RCTs evaluating the role of stereotactic radiosurgery in the management of brain metastases and these have been included in the neuro-oncology chapter (Andrews *et al.*, 2004; Aoyama *et al.*, 2006).

Andrews DW, Scott CB, Sperduto PW, Flanders AE, Gaspar LE, Schell MC, Werner-Wasik M, Demas W, Ryu J, Bahary JP, Souhami L, Rotman M, Mehta MP, Curran WJ Jr. Whole brain radiation therapy with or without stereotactic radiosurgery boost for patients with one to three brain metastases: phase III results of the RTOG 9508 randomised trial. *Lancet* 2004; **363**: 1655–1672.

Aoyama H, Shirato H, Tago T, Nakagawa K, Toyoda T, Hatano K, Kenjyo M, Oya N, Hirota S, Shioura H, Kunieda E, Inomata T, Hayakawa K, Katoh N, Kobashi G. Stereotactic radiosurgery plus whole-brain radiation therapy vs stereotactic radiosurgery alone for the treatment of brain metastases – a randomised controlled trial. *JAMA* 2006; **21**: 2483–2491.

Aziz TZ, Peggs D, Sambrook MA, Crossman AR. Lesion of the subthalamic nucleus for the alleviation of 1-methyl-4-phenyl-1,2,3,6-tetrahydropyridine (MPTP)-induced parkinsonism in the primate. *Mov Disord* 1991; **6**: 288–292.

Ballantyne HT Jr, Cassidy WL, Flanagan NB, Marino R Jr. Stereotaxic anterior cingulotomy for neuropsychiatric illness and intractable pain. *J Neurosurg* 1967; **26**: 488–495.

Ben-Menachem E, Mañon-Espaillat R, Ristanovic R, Wilder BJ, Stefan H, Mirza W, Tarver WB, Wernicke JF. Vagus nerve stimulation for treatment of partial seizures: 1. A controlled study of effect on seizures. First International Vagus Nerve Stimulation Study Group. *Epilepsia* 1994; **35**: 616–626.

Bergman H, Wichmann T, DeLong MR. Reversal of experimental parkinsonism by lesion of the subthalamic nucleus. *Science* 1990; **249**: 1436–1438.

Bittar RG, KarPurkayastha I, Owen SL, Bear RE, Green A, Wang SY, Aziz TZ. Deep brain stimulation for pain relief: a meta-analysis. *J Clin Neurosci* 2005; **12**: 515–519.

Burcktkhardt G. Uber rindexcision, als beitrag zur operativen therapie der psychosen. *Allg Z Psyhciatr Med* 1891; **47**: 463–548.

Engel J. Finally, a randomised, controlled trial of epilepsy surgery. *N Engl J Med* 2001; **345**: 365–366.

Freeman W. Transorbital leucotomy. *Lancet* 1948; **2**: 371–373.

Handforth A, DeGiorgio CM, Schachter SC, Uthman BM, Naritoku DK, Tecoma ES, Henry TR, Collins SD, Vaughn BV, Gilmartin RC, Labar DR, Morris GL 3rd, Salinsky MC, Osorio I, Ristanovic RK, Labiner DM, Jones JC, Murphy JV, Ney GC, Wheless JW. Vagus nerve stimulation therapy for partial-onset seizures: a randomized active-control trial. *Neurology* 1998; **51**: 48–55.

Horsley V, Clarke RH. The structure and functions of the cerebellum examined by a new method. *Brain* 1908; **31**: 45–124.

Krack P, Batir A, Van Blercom N, Chabardes S, Fraix V, Ardouin C, Koudsie A, Limousin PD, Benazzouz A, LeBas JF, Benabid AL, Pollak P. Five-year follow-up of bilateral stimulation of the sub-thalamic nucleus in advanced Parkinson's disease. *N Engl J Med* 2003; **349**: 1925–1934.

Kupsch A, Benecke R, Müller J, Trottenberg T, Schneider GH, Poewe W, Eisner W, Wolters A, Müller JU, Deuschl G, Pinsker MO, Skogseid IM, Roeste GK, Vollmer-Haase J, Brentrup A, Krause M, Tronnier V, Schnitzler A, Voges J, Nikkhah G, Vesper J, Naumann M, Volkmann J; Deep-Brain Stimulation for Dystonia Study Group. Pallidal deep-brain stimulation in primary generalijzed or segmental dystonia. *N Engl J Med* 2006; **355**: 1978–1990.

Leksell L. The stereotactic method and radiosurgery of the brain. *Acta Chir Scand* 1951; **107**: 316–319.

Leksell L. Stereotactic radiosurgery. *J Neurol Neurosurg Psychiatry* 1983; **46**: 797–803.

Mashour GA, Walker EE, Martuza RL. Psychosurgery: past, present, and future. *Brain Res Rev* 2005; **48**: 409–419.

Mayberg HS, Lozano AM, Voon V, McNeely HE, Seminowicz D, Hamani C, Schwalb JM, Kennedy SH. Deep brain stimulation for treatment-resistant depression. *Neuron* 2005; **45**: 651–660.

Moniz E. Essai d'in traitement chirurgical de certaine psychoses. *Bull Acad Med* 1937; **93**: 1379–1385.

Pollock BE. An evidence-based medicine review of stereotactic radiosurgery. *Prog Neurol Surg* 2006; **19**: 152–170.

Spiegel EA, Wycis HT, Marks M, Lee AJ. Stereotaxic apparatus for operations on human brain. *Science* 1947; **106**: 349–350.

Weaver FM, Follett K, Stern M, Hur K, Harris C, Marks WJ Jr, Rothlind J, Sagher O, Reda D, Moy CS, Pahwa R, Burchiel K, Hogarth P, Lai EC, Duda JE, Holloway K, Samii A, Horn S, Bronstein J, Stoner G, Heemskerk J, Huang GD; CSP 468 Study Group. Bilateral deep brain stimulation vs best medical therapy for patients with advanced Parkinson disease: a randomized controlled trial. *JAMA* 2009; **301**: 63–73.

Wiebe S, Blume WT, Girvin JP, Eliasziw M. Effectiveness and Efficiency of Surgery for Temporal Lobe Epilepsy Study Group. A randomized, controlled trial of surgery for temporal-lobe epilepsy. *N Engl J Med* 2001; **345**: 311–318.

5.1 Surgery for temporal lobe epilepsy

Details of study

This study by the Effectiveness and Efficiency of Surgery for Temporal Lobe Epilepsy Group is the first placebo-controlled randomized trial (PRCT) to assess the efficacy and safety of surgical treatment for temporal lobe epilepsy. The study was carried out at the London Health Sciences Center, University of Western Ontario, Canada.

Study references

Main study

Wiebe S, Blume WT, Girvin JP, Eliasziw M. Effectiveness and Efficiency of Surgery for Temporal Lobe Epilepsy Study Group. A randomized, controlled trial of surgery for temporal lobe epilepsy. *N Engl J Med* 2001; **345**: 311–318.

Related reference

Engel J Jr. The timing of surgical intervention for mesial temporal lobe epilepsy: a plan for a randomised controlled clinical trial. *Arch Neurol* 1999; **56**: 1338–1341.

Study design

- PRCT

Class of evidence	I
Randomization	Medical treatment versus surgery
Number of patients	80
Follow-up	Primary outcomes: 1 year
	Secondary outcomes: None
Number of centres	1
Stratification	Presence or absence of generalized motor seizures

- Patients randomized to medical treatment were put on a 1-year waiting list for surgery (the standard practice in the study centre).

- Patients randomized to surgery were admitted for pre-operative evaluation within 48 h of randomization.

- Of the 86 eligible patients, 80 agreed to participate with 40 randomized to each arm of the trial.

- Analysis was performed on an intention-to-treat basis.

Outcome measures

Primary endpoint

- Freedom from seizures impairing awareness (i.e. disabling seizures) at 1 year

Other endpoints analysed

- Freedom from all seizures, including auras.
- Frequency of seizures in those that were not seizure-free was analysed by calculating percentage change in monthly average.
- Mean severity of all seizures assessed at 3-monthly intervals using the Liverpool Seizure Severity Scale that scores the severity from 10 to 48 with higher scores reflecting increased severity.
- Quality of life was assessed using a standard epilepsy quality of life inventory (QOLIE-89) that scores quality of life from 0 to 100 with higher score reflecting superior quality of life.
- Number of patients employed or attending school was recorded at 3-monthly intervals.

Results

- 100% follow-up with no cross-overs.

Outcome	Surgery group	Medical group	Statistical significance
Freedom from disabling seizures	58% free	8% free	$p < 0.001$
Freedom from all seizures	38% free	3% free	$p < 0.001$
Change in frequency of disabling seizures	100%	34%	$p < 0.001$
Mean severity of residual seizures (Scale = 10–48)	21.4	26.5	No significant difference
Mean quality of life from 3 to 12 months (Scale 0–100)	72	59	$p < 0.001$
Percentage employed or attending school at 1 year	56.4	38.5	No significant difference

- Four patients in surgical group did not undergo surgery but of those who did undergo surgery 64% were free from disabling seizures and 42% were free from all seizures.
- One patient in the medical group died from sudden unexplained causes.
- Four patients had adverse affects from surgery: one patient with wound infection; one with sensory disturbance in one lower limb secondary to a focal thalamic infarct; and two with verbal memory disturbance affecting occupation.
- Depression occurred in 18% of patients in the surgical group and in 20% of patients in the medical group.

Conclusions

Surgery for temporal lobe epilepsy is not only safe but also superior to prolonged medical treatment.

Critique

The study by Wiebe *et al.* showed that RCTs of surgery for epilepsy are feasible. In addition, the trial showed that surgery for temporal lobe epilepsy is safe and effective. The follow-up time of the trial had to be limited to 1 year as all patients entered into the trial would ultimately undergo surgery, although those randomized to the medical arm would go on the 1-year waiting list. Indeed, it was this 1-year waiting list that allowed the ethical randomization of patients and allowed the trial to be undertaken. Even with this short period of follow-up the authors were able to show a statistically significant difference between the two treatment arms.

Several criticisms have been levied against the trial including the outcome assessments used. For example, the questionnaires used to assess outcome may not have picked up on subtle personality changes following the resection of amygdala and hippocampus. However, the authors of the trial have indicated that patients undergoing surgery rated themselves better than the medically treated patients on functions that would be affected by the loss of the amygdala and hippocampus including memory and emotional well-being. Although questions have been raised regarding the antiepileptic medication used to try to control seizures in patients in the medical arm of the trial, Wiebe and colleagues have emphasized that all patients were given optimal doses and medication combinations by experienced epilepsy specialists. This trial has confirmed that there is a role of surgery for medically refractory epilepsy. It is estimated that, at least in the United States, approximately only 1.5% of eligible patients undergo surgery for epilepsy control (Engel and Shewmon, 1993). It remains to be seen whether the number of people undergoing surgery will increase as a result of this trial. Certainly, the future of surgical treatment has been secured and there is also interest in radiosurgery and DBS to treat epilepsy.

Engel J Jr, Shewmon DA. Overview: who should be considered a surgical candidate? In: Engel J Jr, ed. Surgical treatment of the epilepsies. 2nd ed. New York: Raven Press, 1993: 23–24.

5.2 **Vagal nerve stimulation for epilepsy**

Details of studies

VNS is now a well-established treatment for refractory epilepsy and a number of efficacy trials have been performed. The trials described in this section are landmarks because they represent the early prospective, randomized studies that changed efficacy studies from a number of case series to Level I evidence and led to the much more widespread use of VNS.

Study references

Main studies

Ben-Menachem E, Mañon-Espaillat R, Ristanovic R, Wilder BJ, Stefan H, Mirza W, Tarver WB, Wernicke JF. Vagus nerve stimulation for treatment of partial seizures: 1. A controlled study of effect on seizures. First International Vagus Nerve Stimulation Study Group. *Epilepsia* 1994; **35**: 616–626.

Handforth A, DeGiorgio CM, Schachter SC, Uthman BM, Naritoku DK, Tecoma ES, Henry TR, Collins SD, Vaughn BV, Gilmartin RC, Labar DR, Morris GL 3rd, Salinsky MC, Osorio I, Ristanovic RK, Labiner DM, Jones JC, Murphy JV, Ney GC, Wheless JW. Vagus nerve stimulation therapy for partial-onset seizures: a randomized active-control trial. *Neurology* 1998; **51**: 48–55.

Related studies

George R, Salinsky M, Kuzniecky R, Rosenfeld W, Bergen D, Tarver WB, Wernicke JF. Vagus nerve stimulation for treatment of partial seizures: 3. Long-term follow-up on first 67 patients exiting a controlled study. First International Vagus Nerve Stimulation Study Group. *Epilepsia* 1994; **35**: 637–643.

Ramsay RE, Uthman BM, Augustinsson LE, Upton AR, Naritoku D, Willis J, Treig T, Barolat G, Wernicke JF. Vagus nerve stimulation for treatment of partial seizures: 2. Safety, side effects, and tolerability. First International Vagus Nerve Stimulation Study Group. *Epilepsia* 1994; **35**: 627–633.

Study designs

	Ben-Menachem *et al.*	Handforth *et al.*
Class of evidence	I	I
Randomization	High versus low stimulation parameters (see below)	High versus low stimulation parameters
Number of patients	83 (67 included in analysis)	254 (196 included in analysis)
Follow-up	14-week period of stimulation (last 12 weeks included in efficacy analysis)	3 months after 2-week 'ramp-up' period where stimulation maximized
Number of centres	17 (12 in United States)	20 (all United States)
Stratification	None	None

◆ Inclusion criteria:

Ben-Menachem *et al*: Medically refractory partial seizures (at least six per month during a 12-week baseline period).

Handforth *et al:* ≥6 partial-onset seizures involving alteration in consciousness (complex partial or secondary generalized) over 30 days with no more than 21 days between seizures; other seizure types; be able to submit accurate seizure counts (or by a carer); 12–65 years; use contraception if female and fertile; be on 1–3 marketed antiepileptic drugs on a stable regimen.

◆ Exclusion criteria:

Ben-Menachem *at al:* A concomitant unstable medical condition; seizure aetiology best treated by another means, e.g. resective surgery; pregnancy.

Handforth *et al:* Deteriorating neurologic or medical conditions; pregnancy; cardiac or pulmonary disease; active peptic ulcer; history of non-epileptic seizures; ≥1 episode of status epilepticus in past 12 months; prior cervical vagotomy; inability to consent; prior VNS; prior DBS; resective epilepsy surgery; inability to perform pulmonary function tests or to attend clinic.

◆ Demographics in the two trials are very similar with mean age around 32–35 years with a range of 13–60 years.

◆ The Ben-Menachem study was a smaller, preliminary RCT that showed VNS is safe and potentially effective in seizure reduction. Handforth *et al.* went on to confirm these results in a larger cohort with a high (99%) completion rate.

Outcome measures

Primary endpoints

Ben-Menachem *et al:* Overall change in seizure frequency for high- and low-frequency groups.

Handforth *et al:* Percentage change in total seizure frequency during treatment period compared to baseline.

Secondary endpoints

Ben-Menachem *et al:*
◆ Changes in seizure intensity and duration
◆ Patient reported ability to 'abort' or 'decrease' a seizure as a result of magnet use
◆ Global ratings by patients, companions and investigators (reported by Ramsay *et al.*, 1994)

Handforth *et al:*
◆ Between-group comparisons of seizures involving alteration of awareness
◆ Within-group changes in seizure frequency during treatment compared to baseline
◆ Number of patients with 50% or 75% seizure frequency reductions
◆ Global evaluation scores
◆ Adverse events

Results

Reduction in seizure frequency was similar in both trials and both trials showed that high-frequency VNS significantly reduces seizures compared to baseline, whereas low-frequency VNS does not. Seizure reduction occurred for both total seizures as well as partial-onset seizures with alteration of awareness. These reductions occurred whether or not the patient had auras. Seizure intensity or duration was not significantly changed. However, regarding all of these results, there was considerable individual variation in response, and although there was a mean reduction in frequency, some patients suffered an increase in seizure frequency with VNS. Global ratings of change indicated significant improvement reported by interviewers but not by the patients or companions. Interestingly, global ratings improved with both high and low stimulation but significantly higher with the former. Side effects of stimulation included voice change, throat paraesthesiae, dyspnoea, and cough. Infection occurred in approximately 11–12% of patients and there were no reported device-related deaths.

	Seizure reduction %		
	High-frequency group	Low-frequency group	*p*-value (between groups)
Ben-Menachem *et al.*	30.9	11.3	0.029
Handforth *et al.*	27.9	15.2	0.02

Conclusions

High-frequency VNS significantly reduces the frequency of seizures in patients with refractory epilepsy.

Critique

Cooper *et al.* were the first to trial brain stimulation for the treatment of epilepsy (Cooper *et al.*, 1973; Cooper *et al.*, 1976; Cooper *et al.*, 1977; Cooper and Upton, 1978). Unfortunately, controlled trials failed to confirm these results (Van Buren *et al.*, 1978: Wright *et al.*, 1984). Several DBS targets have been used to treat epilepsy including the hippocampus (Velasco *et al.*, 2000), the caudate nucleus (Chkhenkeli *et al.*, 1997), and the centromedian thalamic nucleus (Fischer *et al.*, 1992; Velasco *et al.*, 1995), and the posterior hypothalamus (Mirski and Fisher, 1994). More recently the STN has been selected as a target for DBS in epilepsy (Benadid *et al.*, 2002). Stephan Chabardes from the Grenoble group is currently overseeing a RCT (STIMEP) to assess the STN as a target in pharmacoresistant epilepsy and the results of the stimulation of the anterior thalamus in epilepsy (SANTE) trial are close to publication at the time of writing. It may be expected that DBS will be more efficacious in seizure reduction than VNS as the stimulation is directly affecting the brain rather than relying on some method of anterograde stimulation. However, there is no doubt that VNS is safer as it doesn't have a risk of stroke.

The landmark studies described here are impressive in that they applied the principles of prospective, randomized drug trials to a surgical treatment and were well executed. They are, however, far from perfect. One of the main problems is the use of a low-frequency stimulation group as a 'placebo'. This was a necessary compromise in order to ensure adequate 'blinding' as those with no stimulation would be aware that they were not receiving it. But it is not as good as a 'true' placebo group. The fact that there was a seizure reduction in this 'placebo' group illustrates this point. A second flaw is that seizure reduction in the first 3 months may underestimate the long-term improvement, as evidence suggests that efficacy improves even up to 18 months after the onset of therapy (Uthman *et al.*, 1993; Salinsky *et al.*, 1996). Despite these criticisms concerning efficacy, both trials established VNS as a safe therapy with beneficial effects, in some patients more than others.

Benadid AL, Minotti L, Koudsié A. de Saint Martin A, Hirsch E. Antiepileptic effect of high-frequency stimulation of the subthalamic nucleus (corpus luysi) in a case of medically intractable epilepsy caused by focal dysplasia: a 30-month follow-up: technical case report. *Neurosurgery* 2002; **50**: 1385–1391.

Chkhenkeli SA, Chkhenkeli IS. Effects of therapeutic stimulation of nucleus caudatus on epileptic electrical activity of brain patients with intractable epilepsy. *Stereotact Funct Neurosurg* 1997; **69**: 221–224.

Cooper IS, Upton AR. Use of chronic cerebellar stimulation for disorders of inhibition. *Lancet* 1978; **1**: 595–560.

Cooper IS, Amin I, Gilman S. The effect of chronic cerebellar stimulation upon epilepsy in man. *Trans Am Neurol Assoc* 1973; **98**: 192–196.

Cooper IS, Amin I, Riklan M, Waltz JM, Poon TP. Chronic cerebellar stimulation in epilepsy. Clinical and anatomical studies. *Arch Neurol* 1976; **33**: 559–570.

Cooper IS, Amin I, Upton A, Riklan M, Watkins S, McLellan L. Safety and efficacy of chronic cerebellar stimulation. *Appl Neurophysiol* 1977; **40**: 124–134.

Fischer RS, Uematsu S, Krauss GL, Cysyk BJ, McPherson R, Lesser RP, Gordon B, Schwerdt P, Rise M. Placebo-controlled pilot study of centromedian thalamic stimulation in treatment of intractable seizures. *Epilepsia* 1992; **33**: 841–851.

Mirski MA, Fisher RS. Electrical stimulation of the mammillary nuclei increases seizure threshold to pentylenetetrazol in rats. *Epilepsia* 1994; **35**: 1309–1316.

Ramsay RE, Uthman BM, Augustinsson LE, Upton AR, Naritoku D, Willis J, *et al.* Vagus nerve stimulation for treatment of partial seizures: 2. Safety, side effects, and tolerability. First International Vagus Nerve Stimulation Study Group. *Epilepsia* 1994; **35**: 627–636.

Salinsky MC, Uthman BM, Ristanovic RK, Wernicke JF, Tarver WB. Vagus nerve stimulation for the treatment of medically intractable seizures. Results of a 1-year open-extension trial. Vagus Nerve Stimulation Study Group. *Archives of Neurology* 1996; **53**: 1176–1180.

Uthman BM, Wilder BJ, Penry JK, Dean C, Ramsay RE, Reid SA, Hammand EJ, Tarver WB, Wernicke JF. Treatment of epilepsy by stimulation of the vagus nerve. *Neurology* 1993; **43**: 1338–1345.

Van Buren JM, Wood JH, Oakley J, Hambrecht F. Preliminary evaluation of cerebellar stimulation by double-blind stimulation and biological criteria in the treatment of epilepsy. *J Neurosurg* 1978; **48**: 407–416.

Velasco F, Velasco M, Velasco AL, Jiminez F, Marquez J, Rise M. Electrical stimulation of the centromedian thalamic nucleus in the control of the seizures: long-term studies. *Epilepsia* 1995; **36**: 63–71.

Velasco M, Velasco F, Velasco AL, Boleaga B, Jimenez F, Brito F, Marquez I. Subacute electrical stimulation of the hippocampus blocks intractable temporal lobe seizures and paroxysmal EEG activities. *Epilepsia* 2000; **41**: 158–169.

Wright GD, McLellan DL, Brice JG. A double-blind trial of chronic cerebellar stimulation in twelve patients with severe epilepsy. *J Neurol Neurosurg Psychiatry* 1984; **47**: 769–774.

5.3 **Pallidal stimulation for dystonia**

Details of study

The first and most important study of DBS for dystonia was carried out by the Deep Brain Stimulation for Dystonia Study Group in Germany, Austria, and Norway between 2002 and 2004. This study evaluated patients with primary generalized or segmental dystonia with bilateral stimulation of the ventral border of the GPi being compared to sham stimulation for the first 3 months after surgery. The study concludes that stimulation leads to a significant clinical improvement.

Study references

Main study

Kupsch A, Benecke R, Müller J, Trottenberg T, Schneider GH, Poewe W, Eisner W, Wolters A, Müller JU, Deuschl G, Pinsker MO, Skogseid IM, Roeste GK, Vollmer-Haase J, Brentrup A, Krause M, Tronnier V, Schnitzler A, Voges J, Nikkhah G, Vesper J, Naumann M, Volkmann J; Deep-Brain Stimulation for Dystonia Study Group. Pallidal deep-brain stimulation in primary generalized or segmental dystonia. *N Engl J Med* 2006; **355**: 1978–1990.

Related Study

Mueller J, Skogseid IM, Benecke R, Kupsch A, Trottenberg T, Poewe W, Schneider GH, Eisner W, Wolters A, Müller JU, Deuschl G, Pinsker MO, Roeste GK, Vollmer-Haase J, Brentrup A, Krause M, Tronnier V, Schnitzler A, Voges J, Nikkhah G, Vesper J, Naumann M, Volkmann J; Deep-Brain Stimulation for Dystonia Study Group. Pallidal deep brain stimulation improves quality of life in segmental and generalized dystonia: results from a prospective, randomized sham-controlled trial. *Mov Disord* 2008; **23**: 131–134.

Study design

- Double-blind, sham-controlled, randomized trial.
- Followed by 6 months of open-label treatment leading to a total of 6 months of stimulation.

Class of evidence	I
Randomization	Neurostimulation versus sham stimulation
Number of patients	40
Follow-up	9 months total (100% follow-up)
	Primary endpoint:
	• Improvement in dystonia at 3 months
	Secondary endpoints:
	• Improvement in dystonia after a further 6 months of open-label treatment
	• Activities of daily living
	• Quality of life
Number of centres	10
Stratification	None

- The Burke–Fahn–Marsden Dystonia Rating Scale (BFMDRS) was significantly lower in the stimulation group.
- Inclusion criteria: 'Marked disability' owing to primary generalized or segmental dystonia; age 14–75 years.
- Exclusion criteria: Surgical contraindications; previous brain surgery; cognitive impairment (<120 on the Mattis Dementia Rating Scale); moderate to Severe Depression (>25 on the Beck depression inventory); marked brain atrophy on CT or MRI.

Outcome measures

Primary endpoint

- Motor score of the BFMDRS at 3 months and after 6 months of continuous stimulation

Secondary endpoints

- Motor score (BFMDRS) after 6 months of continuous stimulation
- Quality of life assessed with the Medical Outcomes Study 36-Item Short Form General Health Survey (SF-36) questionnaire
- Activities of Daily Living and Disability Score on the BFMDRS
- Various other 'exploratory endpoints' also analysed, e.g. severity of dystonia and pain using a visual analogue score, and rate of response (defined as an improvement in motor scores of >25%)

Results

Neurostimulation versus sham stimulation

- 3 months follow-up.

	Stimulation group	Sham group	Statistical significance
Improvement in motor scores	39.3%	4.9%	$p < 0.001$
Improvement in disability scores	37.5%	8.3%	$p < 0.001$
Percentage of patients with a positive response to treatment (>25% improvement in motor score)	75%	15%	$p < 0.001$
Improvement in physical component of SF-36	29.8%	3.8%	$p = 0.02$

- Neurostimulation was significantly better in all symptom subscores of the BFMDRS and most of the disability scores.

Open-label extension

- Further improvements occurred, although the extra 3 months in the stimulated group did not produce significant changes.

- Motor improvements were seen in the majority of patients: ≥75% improvement (16.7% of patients); ≥50% improvement (45% of patients); and ≥25% improvement (75% of patients).

Other findings

- Drug use and depression also decreased in the stimulation group.
- The most important adverse event was implant infection.

Conclusions

Neurostimulation of the GPi is an effective treatment for both primary generalized and segmental dystonia.

Critique

Sham-controlled surgical trials are relatively rare but neurostimulation lends itself to these types of trials as the sham group can still cross-over to stimulation after the comparison period is over. This was one of the first trials of this nature in functional neurosurgery. Dystonia is a rare condition that is generally not very responsive to medical treatment. Initial case series of neurostimulation for dystonia looked encouraging. There are two factors that make a randomized trial more difficult. Firstly, the numbers are small. Therefore, the benefit has to be great to get statistical significance of any difference. This trial was powered on the basis that 40 patients would be needed to show a 25% difference (90% power) with a 10% drop out rate and a 5% error. The other problem is that the effects of neurostimulation on the GPi are slow to act. It is very rare to get an instantaneous response (other than side effects), and in some patients it can take months to get full benefit from stimulation. One criticism is, therefore, that it is possible that if the study period was longer, an even greater difference may have been demonstrated. Another criticism is that there were positive responses in the sham (control) group (three patients). If the improvement is due to stimulation, why should this be the case? One possibility is the 'stun' or lesional effect of electrode implantation that is certainly seen in subthalamic stimulation for PD. A final criticism is that this trial involved both segmental and generalized dystonias rather than a single entity. The pathophysiology of dystonia is poorly understood and therefore this may not be a valid criticism.

This was the first major randomized trial in functional neurosurgery. Although many centres practised neurostimulation for dystonia before this study, it has provided adequate justification for the continuing use of this technique.

5.4 **Subthalamic nucleus stimulation for Parkinson's disease**

Details of study

The STN was identified as a surgical target for the control of symptoms of PD as the result of findings in preclinical primate research. Three studies are considered here. The first is a landmark as it was the first large follow-up study evaluating the efficacy of STN DBS in PD after 5 years and was carried out between 1993 and 1997 in Grenoble, France (Krack *et al.*, 2003). The second is a randomized pairs trial carried out between 2001 and 2004 in Germany and Austria comparing STN DBS plus medical management with best medical management (Deuschl *et al.*, 2006). The third is the first published RCT of DBS versus best medical therapy for advanced PD (Weaver *et al.*, 2009).

Study references

Main studies

Krack P, Batir A, Van Blercom N, Chabardes S, Fraix V, Ardouin C, Koudsie A, Limousin PD, Benazzouz A, LeBas JF, Benabid AL, Pollak P. Five-year follow-up of bilateral stimulation of the subthalamic nucleus in advanced Parkinson's disease. *N Engl J Med* 2003; **349**: 1925–1934.

Deuschl G, Schade-Brittinger C, Krack P, Volkmann J, Schäfer H, Bötzel K, Daniels C, Deutschländer A, Dillmann U, Eisner W, Gruber D, Hamel W, Herzog J, Hilker R, Klebe S, Kloss M, Koy J, Krause M, Kupsch A, Lorenz D, Lorenzl S, Mehdorn HM, Moringlane JR, Oertel W, Pinsker MO, Reichmann H, Reuss A, Schneider GH, Schnitzler A, Steude U, Sturm V, Timmermann L, Tronnier V, Trottenberg T, Wojtecki L, Wolf E, Poewe W, Voges J; German Parkinson Study Group, Neurostimulation Section. A randomized trial of deep-brain stimulation for Parkinson's disease. *N Engl J Med* 2006; **355**: 896–908.

Weaver FM, Follett K, Stern M, Hur K, Harris C, Marks WJ Jr, Rothlind J, Sagher O, Reda D, Moy CS, Pahwa R, Burchiel K, Hogarth P, Lai EC, Duda JE, Holloway K, Samii A, Horn S, Bronstein J, Stoner G, Heemskerk J, Huang GD; CSP 468 Study Group. Bilateral deep brain stimulation vs best medical therapy for patients with advanced Parkinson disease: a randomized controlled trial. *JAMA* 2009; **301**: 63–73.

Related references

Aziz TZ, Peggs D, Sambrook MA, Crossman AR. Lesion of the subthalamic nucleus for the alleviation of 1-methyl-4-phenyl-1,2,3,6-tetrahydropyridine (MPTP)-induced parkinsonism in the primate. *Mov Disord* 1991; **6**: 288–292.

Ballantyne HT Jr, Cassidy WL, Flanagan NB, Marino R Jr. Stereotaxic anterior cingulotomy for neuro-psychiatric illness and intractable pain. *J Neurosurg* 1967; **26**: 488–495.

Bergman H, Wichmann T, DeLong MR. Reversal of experimental parkinsonism by lesion of the subthalamic nucleus. *Science* 1990; **249**: 1436–1438.

Witt K, Daniels C, Reiff J, Krack P, Volkmann J, Pinsker MO, Krause M, Tronnier V, Kloss M, Schnitzler A, Wojtecki L, Bötzel K, Danek A, Hilker R, Sturm V, Kupsch A, Karner E, Deuschl G. Neuropsychological and psychiatric changes after deep brain stimulation for Parkinson's disease: a randomised, multicentre study. *Lancet Neurol* 2008; **7**: 605–614.

Grenoble 5-year follow-up study

Study design

♦ Follow-up study of a surgical series

Class of evidence	III
Randomization	None
Number of patients	49
Length of follow-up	5 years
	Primary endpoints:
	♦ Activities of daily living
	♦ Motor examination
	Secondary endpoints:
	♦ Tremor, rigidity, limb akinesia, speech, postural stability, gait, dyskinesia
	♦ Neuropsychological testing
	♦ Depression and dementia assessments
	♦ Dopaminergic medication dosage
	♦ Requirements
	♦ Stimulation settings
Number of centres	1
Stratification	None

♦ This was the first major paper looking at outcome of STN stimulation in PD with long-term follow-up.

♦ Forty-nine consecutive patients were assessed (there is no control group).

♦ It is important to look at results both 'on' and 'off' medication. Good results 'off' medication can lead to reduction in levodopa and, therefore improvements, in levodopa side effects such as dyskinesias.

♦ This study documents the adverse effects of STN stimulation, in particular the adverse neuropsychological effects that have led some clinicians to prefer globus pallidus DBS.

♦ Inclusion criteria: Clinical diagnosis of PD; severe levodopa-related complications despite optimal medication; age <70 years; bilateral STN stimulation intended.

♦ Exclusion criteria: Surgical contraindications to DBS (e.g. pacemaker); dementia or psychiatric illness.

Outcome measures

Primary endpoints

♦ Scores on Part II (activities of daily living) and part III (motor scores) on the Unified Parkinson's Disease Rating Scale (UPDRS) at 1, 3, and 5 years

Secondary endpoints

♦ Subscores on part III (limb tremor, limb rigidity and limb akinesia, speech, postural stability, and gait) and part IV (dyskinesias) on the UPDRS

- Schwab and England scale of Activities of Daily Living
- Neuropsychological tests
- Mattis dementia rating scale
- Beck depression inventory
- Dose of dopaminergic treatment
- Stimulation settings

Results

On average, patients had a disease duration of 14.6 years. With stimulation in the 'off' medication state, the total part III (motor) UPDRS score improved by 66% at 1 year, 59% at 3 years and 54% at 5 years. At 5 years, tremor improved by 75%, rigidity by 71%, and akinesia by 49%. Speech initially improved but returned to baseline at 5 years. Postural stability and gait also improved. Activities of daily living (part II UPDRS) improved by 66% at 1 year, 51% and 49% at 3 and 5 years respectively (this reduction at 5 years being significant). Five years after surgery, the Schwab and England score showed that most patients were independent (73%) compared to most being dependent on a carer pre-operatively (33% independent). The incidence of painful dystonia 'off' medication also dramatically reduced after surgery. There was generally worsening in the 'on' medication scores with stimulation, as expected. There was no change in the depression scores, but dementia scores worsened over the 5 years. The authors put this down to deterioration due to the degenerative nature of the disease. Probably the most significant results are that levodopa requirement reduced from a mean of 1409 mg at baseline to 518 mg at 5 years ($p < 0.001$). Eleven patients were able to stop levodopa altogether. Adverse events included three deaths (one intracranial haemorrhage, one myocardial infarction 11 months after surgery, and one suicide 6 months after surgery). Other adverse events included dementia and weight gain.

Conclusions

Bilateral STN DBS in Parkinson's disease results in marked improvement in motor function while patients are 'off' medication and in dyskinesia while 'on' medication.

Germany/Austria randomized pairs trial (Deuschl *et al.*, 2006)

Study design

- Multi-centre unblinded randomized pairs trial

Class of evidence	I
Randomization	Bilateral STN DBS + medical therapy versus best medical treatment
Number of patients	156
Length of follow-up	6 months
	Primary endpoints: • Quality of life • Severity of symptoms

	Secondary endpoints: ◆ Dyskinesia ◆ Activities of daily living ◆ Neuropsychiatric function ◆ Health-related quality of life ◆ Adverse events
Number of centres	10
Stratification	None

◆ Inclusion criteria: PD for at least 5 years; <75 years of age; activities of daily living impaired by motor symptoms or dyskinesias despite optimal medical therapy; informed consent.

◆ Exclusion criteria: Dementia; psychiatric symptoms; contraindications to surgery.

◆ Patients enrolled in pairs with randomization to each arm of the trial within 6 weeks.

◆ Analysis was on an intention-to-treat basis.

Outcomes

Primary endpoints

◆ All primary endpoints were calculated as changes from baseline to 6 months.

◆ Quality of life assessed by Parkinson's disease questionnaire (PDQ-39).

◆ Severity in symptoms assessed by Unified Parkinson's Disease Rating Scale Part III (UPDRS-III) while the patients were not 'on' medication.

Secondary endpoints

◆ Dyskinesia and activities of daily living assessed using the Unified Parkinson's Disease Rating Scale Part II (UPDRS-II).

◆ Neuropsychiatric function: Montgomery and Asberg Depression Rating Scale and the Brief Psychiatric Rating Scale.

◆ Health-related quality of life assessed using Medical Outcomes Study 36-item Short-Form General Health Survey (SF-36).

	Outcome favoured STN DBS	Outcome favoured best medical Rx	No difference in the pairs	Statistical significance
Quality of life	64%	36%	0%	$p = 0.02$
Severity of symptoms	71%	27%	3%	$p < 0.001$

Results

◆ An additional analysis on a per-protocol basis gave a favoured outcome in terms of quality of life to 75% of the STN DBS patients versus 25% for the best medical management group ($p < 0.001$).

- STN DBS was associated with a 25% improvement in the PDQ-39 summary index and a 22% improvement in the SF-36 score.
- Activities of daily living were improved by 39% in the STN DBS group but only by 5% in the best medical management group.
- Dyskinesia improved in the STN DBS group but not in the best medical management group.
- Adverse events were significantly greater in the DBS STN group (12.8%) compared to the best medical management group (3.8%, $p = 0.04$).
- There were three deaths in the DBS STN group: one due to an intracerebral haematoma; one from pneumonia; and one suicide.
- There was one death in the best medical group from a motor vehicle accident while driving during a psychotic episode.

Conclusion

DBS STN resulted in a significant and meaningful improvement in quality of life compared to best medical management.

Veterans affairs and University Hospitals US trial (Weaver *et al.*)

Study design

- PRCT of DBS versus best medical therapy

Class of evidence	I
Randomization	Non-blinded DBS versus medical. DBS further randomized into GPi or STN (patients blinded to stimulation site).
Number of patients	255 (134 medical, 60 STN, 61 GPi)
Length of follow-up	6 Months
	Primary endpoint:
	• Time spent in 'on' state without disabling dyskinesias
	Secondary endpoints:
	• Motor function
	• Quality of life
	• Neurocognitive function
	• Adverse events
Number of centres	13
Stratification	• Study site
	• Patient age (<70 versus ≥70 years)

- This was the first large, multi-centre, randomized controlled, blinded trial comparing risks and benefits of DBS versus best medical therapy.
- Comparison of GPi versus STN targets expected after 2 years follow-up.

- DBS significantly improved duration of 'on' time without troubling dyskinesias (4.6 h/day) although there were a significant number of adverse events, greater in the DBS group.
- Inclusion criteria: Idiopathic PD Hoehn and Yahr ≥ Stage 2 'off' medication; responsive to levodopa; persistent disabling symptoms despite medication (e.g. motor fluctuations, dyskinesia); ≥ 3/24 h poor symptom control; stable medical therapy ≥1 month; ≥21 years of age.
- Exclusion criteria: Atypical syndromes; previous surgery for PD; contraindications to surgery; active alcohol or drug abuse; dementia; pregnancy.

Outcome measures

Primary endpoint

- Baseline to 6-month change in time spent in the 'on' state without troubling dyskinesia

Secondary endpoints

- Hoehn and Yahr and Schwab and England scales
- Stand–walk–sit test
- UPDRS
- PDQ-39
- Medication usage
- Neurocognitive battery including; Mattis Dementia Rating Scale, Standardized tests of attention, memory, verbal, executive functioning, language
- 'On' and 'off' time assessed by self-report motor diaries
- Adverse events

Results

The baseline characteristics did not differ between groups except the best medical therapy patients were treated with PD medications for longer (12.6 versus 10.8 years, $p = 0.01$) and had a lower working memory index (97.3 versus 101.2, $p = 0.02$). DBS patients gained 4.6 h/day of 'on' time without troubling dyskinesia compared to 0 h/day in the medical arm ($p < 0.001$). 'Off' time decreased by 2.4 h/day in the DBS group compared to 0 h in the medical arm ($p < 0.001$). Similar changes were experienced by patients over 70 years of age. Motor function improved by 12.3 points in the DBS group (in the 'off' medication state) compared to 1.7 in the medical arm ($p < 0.001$). Activities of daily living and complications of therapy were also significantly better in the DBS group. Stand–walk–sit test improved by 9 s in the DBS group compared to a 0.2 s worsening at 6 months in the medical arm ($p = 0.046$). Medications decreased by 296 mg levodopa equivalent in the DBS group and increased in the medical arm. Quality of life improved in seven of eight sections of the PDQ-39 subscales in the DBS group whereas there was little change in the medical arm. Some of the neurocognitive measures showed slight but significant worsening in the DBS group (working memory, processing speed, phonemic fluency and delayed recall on the Brief Visuospatial Memory Test). However, there were no significant differences on the scales of depression, dementia, and most of the measures assessing language, executive functioning and learning and memory functioning. Regarding adverse events, the DBS group received a significantly greater number of falls, gait disturbance, depression, and dystonia. In the DBS group, surgical site infection was 9.9% and surgical site pain 9.0%. One DBS patient died as a result of cerebral haemorrhage related to the procedure. The overall incidence risk of a serious adverse event was 3.8 times higher in the DBS group and these included psychiatric disorders. However 99% of these were resolved at 6 months.

Conclusions

DBS is more effective than best medical therapy in alleviating disability in moderate to severe PD patients with levodopa-responsive motor complications and no significant cognitive impairment.

Critique

PD is a degenerative condition and available medications are aimed at symptomatic control with none being available to reverse the ongoing neuronal loss. DBS is intended to improve the symptoms of the disease and therefore improve quality of life. The identification of the STN as a target for DBS in the treatment of PD was the direct result of findings in primate models (Bergman et al., 1990; Aziz et al., 1991). Pollak et al. were the first to report STN DBS for the treatment of a patient with PD (Pollak et al., 1993). Although there are many studies looking at STN stimulation in PD, the study by Krack et al. is the longest proof-of-principle follow-up study carried out. The trial by Deuschl et al. was the first study comparing DBS plus medication to medical therapy alone, and the Weaver study is the largest to date and the first to randomize patients to DBS versus best medical therapy. This latter study also stands out among the literature because the clinical outcome was measured by blinded neurologists and because of the extensive quality of life and neuropsychological data measured. The UK 'PDSurg' trial is currently underway with patients being randomized over the first 12 months as to whether the neurostimulators are activated or not. The results of this trial are also eagerly awaited.

Krack et al. showed that bilateral STN stimulation is an effective treatment for all of the motor parts of the UPDRS score 'off' medication, except speech. It allows patients to significantly reduce their dopaminergic medication and therefore reduces the incidence and severity of dyskinesias. There are few adverse effects, but significantly, dementia appears to be increased, irreversibly in two patients. There is also an increase in other neuropsychiatric symptoms with stimulation, including hypomania and depression. In the Weaver study, there was an increase in depression, confusion, and anxiety in the DBS group but it should be noted that these neuropsychiatric complications also occur in the medical group and that the increases were small.

STN stimulation is generally used in the situation where the patient already responds to levodopa (as it has a similar effect) and is not effective if the patient is levodopa unresponsive. Therefore the aim of stimulation is to allow a reduction in medication and an improvement in the side effects—mainly the disabling dyskinesias that occur in the 'on' state. The study by Krack *et al.* showed that STN stimulation significantly improves the motor symptoms of PD, leads to medication reduction and improvements in the activities of daily living. The main limitation of the study is the lack of any randomization and so it is not possible to say whether STN stimulation is better than medication, as there is no official control arm. The rationale for proposing that STN stimulation represents an improvement over medication is that the investigators are able to study the patients 'off' all treatment (drugs and medication). Another criticism is that the assessments were unblinded. In a single group, this could lead to recorder bias. Nevertheless, this study represents the best long-term outcome data available to date. Another important factor that should be borne in mind when considering the results of this study is that when the study was started there was a tendency to operate on younger patients with severe disease.

The trial by Deuschl *et al.* stands out as a landmark in neurostimulation studies for being the first 'large' randomized trial in this area. Although the trial may be criticized for being unblinded, the authors indicate that the need to adjust medication regimens in DBS patients makes it impossible to carry out a blinded study with placebo stimulation. The use of sham surgery was deemed unethical because of the potential complications. The use of a paired analysis allowed relatively small numbers of patients in order to obtain adequate power and it is nonetheless a well-designed and well-executed study. It is of note that the authors chose not to use motor function as a primary outcome and instead used quality of life. The efficacy of DBS needs to account for not only motor function, but neurobehavioural effects, adverse effects, and surgical complications, all of which affect quality of life. The authors of the trial went on to evaluate the neurobehavioural effects at 6 months in 60 patients receiving STN DBS and 63 patients receiving best medical management (Witt *et al.*, 2008). A wide range of neuropsychiatric tests were used and the primary outcome chosen was cognitive functioning. Secondary outcomes included effects on neurobehavioural variables (executive functioning, depression, anxiety, manic symptoms) and quality of life. Although there appeared to be a selective decrease in frontal executive functioning and verbal fluency, the authors concluded that these did not affect quality of life.

The study by Weaver *et al.*, stands out for the reasons given above—i.e. the size of the study, rigorous randomization, blinded assessments, and detailed neuropsychological outcomes. This study has conclusively demonstrated that DBS improves motor outcome without disabling dyskinesias at a small cost of minor dysexecutive functions but that these are limited to certain categories such as working memory and phonemic fluency, they do not affect quality of life. Probably the most useful aspect of this study is the reporting of adverse events that were much higher in the DBS group. Although the majority of these were resolved at 6 months, there was one death related to cerebral haemorrhage. Despite this, it is difficult to comment on death rates in series less than 1000 as the reported death rates in DBS are around 0.5–1% in previous studies. An important aspect of this trial is the inclusion of GPi patients in a randomized fashion, and the results of GPi versus STN as a target in PD will be very interesting.

The potential neuropsychological and psychiatric sequalae of DBS of the STN have been a source of controversy and concern. However, early series of patients undergoing STN DBS revealed inconsistent effects on cognition and neuropsychological sequalae. A comprehensive review of the literature by Woods et al. found that the most common findings were increased verbal fluency and improvements in self-reported symptoms of depression: approximately 69% of studies including scores of verbal fluency reported a significant post-operative reduction (Woods et al., 2002). There was no consistency in reports on post-operative changes in frontal/executive function, cognition, memory or attention and it appears that changes in these modalities occur in 1–2% of patients only (Woods et al., 2002). However, cognitive deficits and mood disturbance appear to be more frequently reported in patients receiving DBS of the STN than in patients undergoing pallidal DBS, a trend that has also been reflected in direct comparisons of these two targets (Walter and Vitek, 2004; Volkmann et al., 2001; Rodriguez-Oroz et al., 2005). Deuschl's group have reported the results of a randomized trial of STN DBS versus best medical management in advanced PD to assess the neuropsychological and psychiatric effects of DBS for Parkinson's (Witt et al., 2008). They found that there was no decline in cognition but there was a selective decrease in frontal cognitive functions.

As DBS has become more widespread, more and older patients are receiving the treatment. The initial anxieties regarding the 'limbic' side effects of stimulation including cognitive decline, behavioural changes, and psychosis (as suggested in the Krack et al. study with the increased incidence of dementia) are becoming more pronounced as later studies have longer follow-up and include older patients. The pendulum that had largely swung towards STN stimulation in favour of globus pallidus stimulation is perhaps starting to swing back, particularly in older patients or those with a hint of psychotic or dementia-related issues. Nonetheless there are still many unanswered questions regarding STN DBS. For example, although DBS has been used when medical therapy has failed, it is possible that the earlier use of neurosurgery may prevent deterioration. Schüpbach et al. carried out a pilot RCT of 20 patients in which 10 were randomized to early bilateral STN DBS and 10 to optimal medical management (Schüpbach et al., 2007). The authors found a statistically significant benefit for DBS in terms of quality of life ($p < 0.05$) and severity of symptoms ($p < 0.001$) over a period of 18 months, thus supporting the idea that there may be potential benefits of STN stimulation as a therapeutic option earlier in Parkinson disease.

STN stimulation has become a popular treatment with over 40,000 implants worldwide. These studies have helped to confirm that it is a useful treatment with lasting effects, but importantly have also identified the negative effects of stimulation. Thus, there are a number of ongoing studies comparing STN to GPi stimulation (including Weaver et al. part two) and other large, randomized trial of DBS such as the 'PDSurg' trial.

Aziz TZ, Peggs D, Sambrook MA, Crossman AR. Lesion of the subthalamic nucleus for the alleviation of 1-methyl-4-phenyl-1,2,3,6-tetrahydropyridine (MPTP)-induced parkinsonism in the primate. *Mov Disord* 1991; **6**: 288–292.

Bergman H, Wichmann T, DeLong MR. Reversal of experimental parkinsonism by lesion of the subthalamic nucleus. *Science* 1990; **249**: 1436–1438.

Pollak P, Benabid AL, Gross C, Gao DM, Laurent A, Benazzouz A, Hoffman D, Gentil M, Perret J. Effects of the stimulation of the subthalamic nucleus in Parkinson disease. *Revue Neurologique* 1993; **149**: 175–176.

Rodriguez-Oroz MC, Obeso JA, Lang AE, Houeto JL, Pollak P, Rehncrona S, Kulisevsky J, Albanese A, Volkmann J, Hariz MI, Quinn NP, Speelman JD, Guridi J, Zamarbide I, Gironell A, Molet J, Pascual-Sedano B, Pidoux B, Bonnet AM, Agid Y, Xie J, Benabid AL, Lozano AM, Saint-Cyr J, Romito L, Contarino MF, Scerrati M, Fraix V, Van Blercom N. Bilateral deep brain stimulation in Parkinson's disease: a multicentre study with 4 years follow-up. *Brain* 2005; **128**: 2240–2249.

Schüpbach WMM, Maltête, D, Houeto JL, Tezenas du Montcel S, Mallet L, Welter ML, Gargiulo M, Béhar C, Bonnet AM, Czernecki V, Pidoux B, Navarro S, Dormont D, Cornu P, Agid Y. Neurosurgery at an earlier stage of Parkinson disease. *Neurology* 2007; **68**: 267–271.

Volkmann J, Allert N, Voges J, Weiss PH, Freund HJ, Sturm V. Safety and efficacy of pallidal or subthalamic nucleus stimulation in advance PD. *Neurology* 2001; **56**: 548–551.

Walter BL, Vitek JL. Surgical treatment for Parkinson's disease. *Lancet Neurol* 2004; **3**: 719–728.

Witt K, Daniels C, Reiff J, Krack P, Volkmann J, Pinsker MO, Krause M, Tronnier V, Kloss M, Schnitzler A, Wojtecki L, Bötzel K, Danek A, Hilker R, Sturm V, Kupsch A, Karner E, Deuschl G. Neuropsychological and psychiatric changes after deep brain stimulation for Parkinson's disease: a randomised, multicentre study. *Lancet Neurol* 2008; **7**: 605–614.

Woods SP, Fields JA, Tröster AI. Neuropsychological sequelae of subthalamic nucleus deep brain stimulation in Parkinson's disease: a critical review. *Neuropsychology Rev* 2002; **12**: 111–126.

5.5 **Pallidal versus STN stimulation for Parkinson's disease**

Details of study

DBS of the GPi has always been a viable alternative to STN stimulation in the treatment of PD. Indeed, some proponents of GPi stimulation have claimed (and still do) that it is a better target than STN for a variety of reasons, but particularly because it is not associated with the limbic or neuropsychiatric complications that can occur with the latter. While many centres have tended to prefer STN as a target, the debate over which is better is now starting to re-emerge. A large, prospective, multi-centre trial would be helpful in this regard, but the small trial described here is a landmark in the sense that it is the only study to date that compares the two in a randomized, prospective fashion and shows that the effects are similar. The main study by Anderson *et al.* is an extension of an earlier study by Burchiel *et al.* (same group) that superseded the previous retrospective studies.

Study references

Main study

Anderson VC, Burchiel KJ, Hogarth P, Favre J, Hammerstad JP. Pallidal vs Subthalamic Nucleus Deep Brain Stimulation in Parkinson Disease. *Arch Neurol* 2005; **62**: 554–560.

Related study

Burchiel K, Anderson VC, Favre J, Hammerstad JP; Comparison of pallidal and subthalamic nucleus deep brain stimulation for advanced Parkinson's disease: Results of a randomized, blinded pilot study. *Neurosurgery* 1999; **45**(6): 1375–82.

Study design

- Double-blind (assessing neurologist and patient), prospective, randomized trial

Class of evidence	I
Randomization	GPi or STN
Number of patients	23 (20 completed 12 months follow-up)
Length of follow-up	12 months
Number of centres	1
Stratification	None

- This is an extension study of the original (Burchiel K *et al.*, 1999 – see above). The original was stopped after 15 patients when the Veteran Affairs/National Institutes of Health launched a multi-centre study of a similar design. That study is still ongoing and results will supersede this one.

- Inclusion criteria: Idiopathic PD (Hoehn and Yahr stage 3–4 'off' medication); 20–80 years of age; prominent bradykinesia and rigidity.

- Exclusion criteria: Surgical contraindications; previous PD surgery; cognitive impairment (<24 on the mini mental state examination or by psychological interview);

depression (>20 on the Beck depression inventory); marked brain atrophy on CT or MRI relative to age; other CNS disease.

- PD severity did not differ between groups at baseline, but STN patients had significantly longer symptom duration than GPi patients (mean 15.6 versus 10.3 years).
- Results showed that STN stimulation had a greater effect on UPDRS improvement ('off' medication motor scores); 48% versus 39%, but this was not significant.

Outcome measures

Primary endpoint

- Change in 'off' medication UPDRS motor score at 12 months

Secondary endpoints

- UPDRS measures of bradykinesia, rigidity, axial symptoms, and dyskinesia rating scale
- Medication use
- Activities of daily living (UPDRS)

Results

UPDRS variable 'off' medication	STN % improved	GPi % improved	p-value
Total motor	48	39	0.40
Rigidity	48	47	0.18
Tremor	89	79	0.51
Bradykinesia	44	33	0.06
Axial symptoms	44	40	0.12
Activities of daily living	28	18	0.48

- Results of stimulation combined with medication were similar, with the only significant difference between GPi and STN being the bradykinesia score.
- Stimulation of either site did not improve 'on' medication scores at 12 months.
- Medication usage reduced by 38% in the STN group compared to 3% in the GPi group ($p = 0.08$).
- Dyskinesia improved in both groups; 89% for GPi and 62% for STN.
- Complications; one intra-operative ischaemic stroke (GPi patient), three subclavicular haematomas (not requiring treatment), one extracranial lead fracture, two STN patients with cognitive complications (one probably related to disease progression).

Conclusions

There are minimal differences to suggest superiority of GPi over STN or vice versa as targets for DBS in PD, although there are individual differences in motor effects between the two nuclei, such as STN being better for bradykinesia and GPI better for 'on' medication dyskinesia.

Critique

This trial can be criticized for a number of reasons including the significant difference in disease duration between the two groups, the variability in recruitment methods in the earlier and follow-up trial, variability in the procedure such as microelectrode recording, and the fact that the patient in the GPi group who suffered an ischaemic stroke was not included in the outcome data. However, it has been considered here as a landmark because it is the first blinded, randomized, prospective trial that brought into question the commonly held belief that STN is a better target than GPi in the treatment of PD. The Veterans Affairs Study by Weaver *et al.* (described above) provided much more data on a larger number of patients. In addition, there are several other large trials comparing the two nuclei that are still awaited at the time of writing. The main criticism of this trial is that the numbers are too small to draw any firm conclusions. This limitation is accepted by the authors who have been involved in the larger study. However, despite the small numbers and lack of significant differences between nuclei, this trial has highlighted the fact that there are differences between the two targets in terms of effects on individual motor symptoms. For example, it would appear that bradykinesia is better improved with STN stimulation, but that the risks of cognitive problems are probably worse (though the small numbers mean that this latter conclusion cannot be confirmed in this study). A second conclusion is that GPi has a better effect on dyskinesia while 'on' medication and that the action of STN to reduce dyskinesias is via its effect on medication reduction. Thus, the implication is that a patient with a low threshold for dyskinesia with less chance of medication reduction may be a good candidate for GPi stimulation. In summary, the trial has highlighted the role of individualizing target selection to each patient.

5.6 Spinal cord stimulation for failed back surgery syndrome

Details of study

Between 10% and 40% of patients who undergo lumbosacral surgery end up with persistent or recurrent chronic neuropathic pain, usually in the legs, known as 'failed back surgery syndrome' (FBSS). Spinal cord stimulation (SCS) has been used to treat FBSS for a number of years and around 35,000 systems are implanted worldwide each year. This is the reason therefore that the PROCESS study reported here (Kumar *et al*, 2007) is a landmark in the field of neuromodulation. It was the first study to report greater pain relief, quality of life, and functional capacity in this patient group. Since the PROCESS study, a 24-month follow-up has also been published that demonstrates long-lasting pain relief.

Study references

Main study

Kumar K, Taylor RS, Jacques L, Eldabe S, Meglio M, Molet J, Thomson S, O'Callaghan J, Eisenberg E, Milbouw G, Buchser E, Fortini G, Richardson J, North RB. Spinal cord stimulation versus conventional medical management for neuropathic pain: a multicentre randomised controlled trial in patients with failed back surgery syndrome. *Pain* 2007; **132**(1–2): 179–188.

Related study

Kumar K, Taylor RS, Jacques L, Eldabe S, Meglio M, Molet J, Thomson S, O'Callaghan J, Eisenberg E, Milbouw G, Buchser E, Fortini G, Richardson J, North RB. The effects of spinal cord stimulation in neuropathic pain are sustained: a 24-month follow-up of the prospective randomized controlled multicenter trial of the effectiveness of spinal cord stimulation. *Neurosurgery* 2008; **63**(4): 762–770.

Study design

• Non-blinded, prospective, randomized, multi-centre trial

Class of evidence	I
Randomization	Spinal cord stimulator versus conventional medical management
Number of patients	100 (88 completed 12 months follow-up)
Length of follow-up	12 months
Number of centres	13
Stratification	None

• This was the first prospective randomized trial comparing SCS plus conventional medical therapy (CMM) to CMM alone.

• The study conclusively demonstrated that SCS improves pain relief and quality of life for FBSS.

• The trial also highlighted the large number of device-related problems that occur in these patients.

• A 12-month follow-up study shows that the improvements persist at 2 years.

- Inclusion criteria: ≥18 years of age; neuropathic radicular pain (L4 and/or L5 and/or S1) predominantly in legs; intensity ≥50/100 mm on VAS; at least 6 months duration; at least one anatomically successful surgery for a herniated disc.
- Exclusion criteria: Another significant or disabling chronic pain condition; perceived inability to receive or operate SCS system; history of coagulation disorder; lupus erythematosus; diabetic neuropathy; rheumatoid arthritis; ankylosing spondylitis; active psychiatric disorder or condition known to affect pain perception; inability to evaluate treatment outcome; life expectancy <1 year; actual or planned pregnancy.

Outcome measures

Primary endpoint

- Proportion of patients achieving at least 50% leg pain relief at 6 months

Secondary endpoints

- 4-day pain diary leg pain (VAS)
- 4-day pain diary back pain (VAS)
- SF-36 Quality of Life Questionnaire
- Oswestry Disability Index
- Morphine and other drug use
- Use of non-drug therapies (e.g. acupuncture or massage)
- Patient satisfaction (satisfied with pain relief, would agree to operation again, and return to work)
- Adverse events

Results

- Primary outcome: 48% of patients in the SCS arm achieved at least 50% pain relief compared to 9% in the medical arm ($p < 0.001$).
- Regarding secondary outcomes, in general, SCS patients improved significantly on most pain and quality of life scores: see table.
- Opioid use was not significantly different between the two groups at 6 months but tended to be less in the SCS group.

Outcome measure	Medical arm	SCS arm	*p*-value
Leg pain relief (≥30%)	18%	64%	<0.0001
Leg pain relief (≥80%)	7%	22%	0.05
SF-36—mean			
Physical function	21.8	38.1	<0.001
Role – physical	8	17.5	0.12
Bodily pain	19.5	33	<0.001
General health	41.3	52.8	<0.001

Outcome measure	Medical arm	SCS arm	p-value
Vitality	31.1	41.3	0.01
Social functioning	33.5	49.3	0.002
Role—emotional	29.5	51.3	0.02
Mental health	50.1	62.6	0.002
Oswestry Disability Index—mean	56.1	44.9	<0.001
Drug therapy			
Opioids	70%	56%	0.20
NSAIDs	50%	34%	0.14
Antidepressants	55%	34%	0.06
Anticonvulsants	50%	26%	0.02
Patient satisfaction			
Satisfied with pain relief	18%	66%	<0.001
Agree with treatment	50%	86%	<0.001
Return to work	3%	11%	0.36

- Cross-over: 28/44 medical patients crossed to SCS at 6 months (plus a further four who failed screening) compared to only five SCS patients who agreed to cross to medical management.

- Complications: 27/84 patients (32%) who received an electrode (either trial or implanted system) experienced 40 device-related complications over 12 months; 20/27, i.e. 24% of the total, required surgery to rectify the problem. Events included electrode migration (10%), infection or wound complications (8%), loss of paraesthesiae (7%). Non-device complications were higher in the medical arm (52% versus 35%) and consisted largely of drug-related events.

Conclusions

Compared with conventional medical therapy alone, SCS improves pain relief, quality of life, functional capacity, and patient satisfaction in selected patients with neuropathic pain related to FBSS.

Critique

The PROCESS study was a well-designed and well-executed trial that represents a landmark because, despite the tens of thousands of SCS systems implanted prior to the trial, efficacy of SCS had not been demonstrated. The main limitation of the trial is that it demonstrates efficacy at 6 months but not in the long term. This can be likened to some of the studies that show lumbar discectomy to be efficacious for short-term (i.e. 6–12 months) pain relief but not over longer periods. However, as a result of the trial there is no doubt that pain is alleviated and that patients are satisfied with the result. Furthermore, the follow-up study looks at 2-year outcomes and goes a long way in answering this question. The trial stands out from many other pain trials in that these measures of patient satisfaction and questions such as whether the patient would have the procedure again are practical questions rather than abstract measures of pain severity.

There have been other RCTs in SCS. For example, Kemler et al. compared SCS plus physical therapy to physical therapy alone and showed that SCS was efficacious (Kemler et al., 2000, 2004, 2006). However, it is notable that all of the patients had previously failed physical therapy and therefore SCS was being compared to a failed treatment. Also, the long-term outcomes showed that the effects of SCS diminished with time. This may be important when analysing the results of the PROCESS study, as outcomes have only been published to 2 years. This 'tolerance' to stimulation has been seen before in studies of DBS for pain (Romanelli and Heit, 2004).

A second RCT and one that is directly relevant to PROCESS was performed by North et al. (2005) comparing reoperation versus SCS in patients with FBSS. This trial had a few problems. For example, there was a high rate of unintended cross-over in both groups (54% reoperation to SCS and 21% the opposite way) and patients receiving worker's compensation were less likely to enter the trial due to lack of insurance authorization.

In summary, the PROCESS study is the first to show that short-term analgesia is better with SCS than medical management in FBSS, although as pointed out by Turner et al. (2007) in their editorial, as there was no sham stimulation, whether the effects were due to 'active' effects of SCS or placebo is difficult to determine.

Kemler MA, Barendse GA, van Kleef M, de Vet HC, Rijks CP, Furnee CA, van den Wildenberg FA. Spinal cord stimulation in patients with chronic reflex sympathetic dystrophy. *N Engl J Med* 2000; **343**: 618–624.

Kemler MA, De Vet HC, Barendse GA, Van Den Wildenberg FA, Van Kleef M. The effect of spinal cord stimulation in patients with chronic reflex sympathetic dystrophy: two years' follow-up of the randomized controlled trial. *Ann Neurol* 2004; **55**: 13–18.

Kemler MA, de Vet HC, Barendse GA, van den Wildenberg FA, van Kleef M. Spinal cord stimulation for chronic reflex sympathetic dystrophy – five-year follow-up. *N Engl J Med* 2006; **354**: 2394–2396.

North RB, Kidd DH, Farrokhi F, Piantadosi SA. Spinal cord stimulation versus repeated lumbosacral spine surgery for chronic pain: a randomized, controlled trial. *Neurosurgery* 2005; **56**: 98–106; discussion 106–107.

Romanelli P, Heit G. Patient-controlled deep brain stimulation can overcome analgesic tolerance. *Stereotact Funct Neurosurg* 2004; **82**: 77–79.

Turner JA, Deyo RA, Loeser JD. Spinal cord stimulation: stimulating questions. *Pain* 2007; **132**: 10–11.

5.7 Deep brain stimulation for treatment-resistant depression

Details of study

This study by Mayberg *et al.* tested the hypothesis that DBS to modulate activity of the grey matter (GM) in area 25 of the cingulate gyrus (Cg25) would produce clinical benefits in patients with treatment-resistant depression. The study was carried out in Toronto, Canada using subgenual cingulate white matter (Cg25WM) as a target in six patients.

Study references

Main study

Mayberg HS, Lozano AM, Voon V, McNeely HE, Seminowicz D, Hamani C, Schwalb JM, Kennedy SH. Deep brain stimulation for treatment-resistant depression. *Neuron* 2005; **45**: 651–660.

Related references

Greenberg BD, Friehs G, Carpenter L, Tyrka A, Malone A, Rezai A, Shapira N, Foote K, Okun M, Goodman W, Rasmussen S, Price L. Deep brain stimulation: clinical findings in intractable depression and OCD. *Neuropsychopharmacology* 2005; **29**: S32.

Mayberg HS, Liotti M, Brannan SK, McGunnis S, Mahurin RK, Jerabek PA, Silva JA, Tekell JL, Martin CC, Fox PT. Reciprocal limbic-cortical function and negative mood: converging PET findings in depression and normal sadness. *Am J Psychiatry* 1999; **156**: 675–682.

Study design

A pilot study to evaluate Cg25WM as a target for DBS in treatment-resistant depression

Class of evidence	III
Randomization	None
Number of patients	6
Follow-up	6 months
	Primary outcomes: Clinical depression Regional cerebral blood flow measurements
	Secondary outcomes: Neuropsychological testing Adverse events
Number of centres	1
Stratification	None

- Inclusion criteria: Treatment-resistant depression; Diagnostic and Statistical Manual of Mental Disorders (DSM-IV) criteria for a major depressive episode of >1 year duration; minimum score of 20 on the Hamilton Depression Rating Scale (HDRS); age <60 years.

- Exclusion criteria: Previous stroke; significant cerebrovascular risk factors; other Axis I psychiatric disorder (e.g. schizophrenia, obsessive-compulsive disorder);

psychotic symptoms; active suicidal intent; recent substance abuse; >60 years of age; inability to comply with follow-up; contraindications to DBS (e.g. cardiac pacemaker).

- Treatment-resistant depression was defined as failure to respond to at least four different classes of antidepressant medication in maximal doses.
- In addition, five out of six patients had failed to respond to electroconvulsive therapy (ECT).

Surgical technique

- Microelectrodes were inserted using a Leksell stereotactic frame.
- Medtronic 3387 quadripolar DBS electrodes were implanted bilaterally.
- Electrode positioning was achieved by MRI mapping: the GM/WM transition area 25 was located at the midpoint between the genu of corpus callosum and the anterior commissure.
- Microelectrode recordings were used to guide insertion into the transitional area between Cg25 (neuronal active area) and Cg25WM (cell sparse area).
- Final electrode positioning was confirmed by post-operative MRI.
- Stimulation parameters were reassessed and adjusted at weekly intervals with increments of 1.0 Volt.
- The mean parameters used were 4.0 Volts with a 60 μs pulse width at a frequency of 130 Hz.

Outcomes

Primary outcomes

- Clinical depression: improvements in depression were monitored using the 17 item HDRS with a clinical response being defined as a reduction of ≥50%
- Regional blood flow: measured using positron emission tomography (PET)

Secondary outcomes

- Neuropsychological testing of cognitive, intellectual, and frontal functioning
- Monitoring of adverse events

Results

Clinical response

- Five out of six patients showed a clinical response (≥50% reduction in HDRS) at 2 months.
- Clinical response was maintained in four out of these five patients at 6 months.

Regional blood flow measurements

- Reduced Cg25WM activity was seen in all patients: both responders and non-responders alike.

• In addition, responders showed an area of hyperactivity in the medial frontal cortex (BA10).

Other findings

• Improvement in early morning sleep disturbance was the earliest sign of a clinical response and was seen in four out of the six patients.

• Improvements were seen in neuropsychological tests.

Adverse effects

• There were no adverse effects on orbitofrontal functioning (such events would be indicative of local DBS adverse effects).

• There were no adverse affective or autonomic effects of increments in stimulator settings.

• All patients experienced psychomotor slowing at higher voltage settings (>7 Volts).

• Two patients received antibiotics for superficial infections related to the connector cables.

Conclusions

Cg25WM is an effective target for DBS in treatment-resistant depression.

Critique

Major depression is the most common psychiatric disorder and depression that is resistant to medication and electroconvulsive therapy is an extremely severe and debilitating condition. In addition to DBS, VNS has also been assessed in the treatment of treatment-resistant depression, and although no randomized trial has been carried out, preliminary studies show some promise (Rush *et al.*, 2000). DBS is still in the exploratory phases for the treatment of this disorder. Greenberg *et al.* noticed improvement in co-morbid depression symptomatology in patients undergoing DBS of the ventral portion of the anterior limb of the internal capsule and the adjacent dorsal ventral striatum for treatment of obsessive-compulsive disorder (Greenberg *et al.*, 2003). The authors then evaluated DBS in the ventral internal capsule in a series of five patients with depression and reported an improvement on the HDRS in all five patients with a mean improvement from 31.4 to 15.8 over 3 months (Greenberg *et al.*, 2005).

The study summarized here by Mayberg *et al.* arose from their previous observations that there was elevated activity of area 25 of the cingulate gyrus (Cg25) in neuroimaging studies of patients with severe treatment-resistant depression (Mayberg *et al.*, 1999). This observation was in concordance with reports of suppression of activity in this same region by antidepressive treatments including selective serotonin reuptake inhibitors (SSRIs) and electroconvulsive therapy. Mayberg *et al.*, therefore, hypothesized that chronic stimulation to modulate Cg25 grey matter may ameliorate symptoms in treatment-resistant depression. The results of their study showed that four out of six patients showed a sustained clinical benefit from DBS of the Cg25WM at 6 months. It should be emphasized that this is a pilot study and Mayberg *et al.* pointed out that, although encouraging, their results are limited by the small sample size, limited follow-up, and the lack of sham surgery or a placebo-control arm. However, Mayberg *et al.* did undertake a trial of blinded DBS discontinuation in one patient and their findings appeared to support Cg25WM stimulation to effect symptom relief. Notwithstanding these difficulties, this study represents a significant landmark in identifying the Cg25WM as a target for DBS in treatment-resistant depression. Also, it is an example of how findings from functional imaging studies have been translated into a novel surgical intervention for a major debilitating disorder.

Greenberg BD, Price LH, Rauch SL, Friehs G, Noren G, Malone D, Carpenter LL, Rezai AR, Rasmussen SA. Neurosurgery for intractable obsessive-compulsive disorder and depression: critical issues. *Neurosurg Clin N Am* 2003; **14**: 199–212.

Rush AJ, George MS, Sackeim HA, Marangell LB, Husain MM, Giller C, Nahas Z, Haines S, Simpsn RK Jr, Goodman R. Vagus nerve stimulation (VNS) for treatment resistant depression: a multicenter study. *Biol Psychiatry* 2000; **47**: 276–286.

5.8 Microvascular decompression for trigeminal neuralgia

The long-term outcome of microvascular decompression (MVD) for trigeminal neuralgia (TN) was established in 1996 with the publication of results of a series of 1185 patients from the Presbyterian University Hospital in Pittsburgh undergoing MVD between 1972 and 1991 (Barker *et al.*, 1996).

Study references

Main study

Barker FG, Janetta PJ, Bissonette DJ, PAC, Larkins MV, Jho HD. The long-term outcome of microvascular decompression for trigeminal neuralgia. *N Engl J Med* 1996; **334**: 1077–1083.

Related study

Janetta PJ. Arterial compression of the trigeminal nerve at the pons in patients with trigeminal neuralgia. *J Neurosurgery* 1967; **26**: 159–162.

Study Design

Class of evidence	II
Randomization	None (see below)
Number of patients	1185
Length of follow-up	>1 year Median 6.2 years 91% at 5 years
Number of centres	1
Stratification	None

- At surgery compressing arteries were separated from the nerve and compressing veins were cauterized and cut.

Outcome measures

Primary endpoints

- Relief of pain: complete relief (excellent outcome) defined as ≥98% pain relief without need for medication; partial relief (good outcome) defined as 75% reduction in pain; failure (poor outcome) defined as recurrence of >25% of pre-operative pain or need for a further surgical procedure.

Secondary endpoints
- Operative findings
- Complications

Results

	Immediately post-op	1 year	10 years
Excellent	82%	75%	64%
Good	16%	9%	4%
Partial	2%	16%	32%

- When repeat surgery was included excellent outcomes were achieved in 80% of patients at 1 year and 70% of patients at 10 years.
- The commonest vessel causing compression was the superior cerebellar artery (75%).
- Venous compression was seen in 68%.
- Complications were uncommon with cerebrospinal fluid (CSF) leak, hearing loss, and facial numbness being the most frequent.
- Recurrence rates were <2% at 5 years and <1% at 10 years.
- Risk factors for recurrence included lack of immediate post-operative relief, female sex, venous compression, and pre-operative symptoms of >8 years duration.

Conclusion

MVD for TN is safe and has a high rate of long-term success.

Critique

MVD of the trigeminal nerve for TN was popularized by Gardner and Janetta (Gardner and Miklos, 1959; Gardner, 1962; Janetta, 1967; Gardner, 1968). Janetta's series considered here is a landmark in the neurosurgical literature as it established the favourable long-term results of MVD. There are various surgical strategies that are available to treat TN including MVD, partial rhizotomy of the sensory root, percutaneous compression (balloon compression), glycerol rhizotomy, radiofrequency thermorhizotomy, and stereotactic radiosurgery. Although there has been no study comparing the long-term effectiveness of these different surgical techniques, a review of the literature of those studies that had at least a 5-year mean follow-up found that MVD has the best reported long-term results (Tatli et al., 2008).

MVD is firmly established as the most successful treatment option for TN refractory to medical therapy. However, there has been substantial debate in the literature regarding the mechanism by which this operation if effective. Walter Dandy is credited in the 1940s with proposing that TN may be caused by compression of the trigeminal nerve by the superior cerebellar artery at its point of entry into the pons. Janetta is credited subsequently with elaborating the concept of pulsatile compression at the root entry zone (REZ), which was defined as a junctional area between central and peripheral myelin (Janetta, 1977; Janetta, 1980). It was postulated that relief of this compression explains the efficacy of MVD. However, Gardner and Miklos had previously stated that the critical component of MVD is manipulation of the nerve itself (Gardner and Miklos, 1959). This observation led to the hypothesis that MVD is effective because of trauma to the nerve itself, a theory that would appear to be supported by the efficacy of partial section of the trigeminal nerve. The most vociferous opponent of Janetta's theory of microvascular compression at the REZ was Adams in Oxford who presented anatomical, clinical, neuropathological, and neurophysiological findings that he proposed supported the hypothesis that trauma to the nerve during dissection and subsequent 'decompensation' of the nerve were more likely to explain the efficacy of MVD (Adams, 1989). The mechanism of MVD efficacy remains to be elucidated. However, more recently Sindou has reported the results of a large series for which clear-cut marked vascular compression at surgery is associated with higher success rates of more than 90% (Sindou *et al.*, 2007).

Adams CBT. Microvascular decompression: an alternative view and hypothesis. *J Neurosurg* 1989; **57**: 1–12.

Gardner WJ. Concerning the mechanism of trigeminal neuralgia and hemifacial spasm. *J Neurosurg* 1962; **19**: 947–958.

Gardner WJ. Trigeminal neuralgia. *Clin Neursurg* 1968; **15**: 1–56.

Gardner WJ, Miklos MV. Response of trigeminal neuralgia and hemifacial spasm. JAMA 1959; **170**: 1773–1776.

Janetta PJ. Treatment of trigeminal neuralgia by suboccipital and transtentorial cranial operations. *Clin Neurosurg* 1977; **24**: 538–549.

Janetta PJ. Neurovascular compression in cranial and systemic disease. *Ann Surg* 1980; **192**: 518–525.

Sindou M, Leston J, Decullier E, Chapus F. Microvascular decompression for primary trigeminal neuralgia: long-term effectiveness and prognostic factors in a series of 362 consecutive patients with clear-cut neurovascular conflicts who underwent pure decompression. *J Neurosurg* 2007; **107**: 1144–1153.

Tatli M, Satici O, Kanpolat Y, Sindou M. Various surgical modalities for trigeminal neuralgia: literature study of respective long-term outcomes. *Acta Neurochir* (Wein) 2008; **150**: 234–255.

5.9 **Neural transplantation for Parkinson's disease**

Details of studies

Neural transplantation for the treatment of neurodegenerative disorders has long been a holy grail for neurosurgeons. The three studies included here are the first post-mortem demonstrations that foetal neural cells grafted into patients with PD can survive and function for over a decade in the host's brain (Li *et al.*, 2008; Kordower *et al.*, 2008; Mendez *et al.*, 2008). Furthermore, they are the first demonstration that, at least in a subset of patients, a fraction of grafted cells develops Lewy body pathology, typical of the host Parkinsonian pathology. These three long-term studies were carried out on three patients in Canada, two patients in the United States, and two patients in Sweden, and were published simultaneously in addition to one of the patients that was reported later (Kordower *et al.*, 2008).

Study references

Main studies

Kordower JH, Chu Y, Hauser RA, Freeman TB, Olanow CW. Lewy body-like pathology in long-term embryonic nigral transplants in Parkinson's disease. *Nat Med* 2008; **14**: 504–506.

Li JY, Englund E, Holton JL, Soulet D, Hagell P, Lees AJ, Lashley T, Quinn NP, Rehncrona S, Bjorklund A, Widner H, Revesz T, Lindvall O, Brundin P. Lewy bodies in grafted neurons in subjects with Parkinson's disease suggest host-to-graft disease propagation. *Nat Med* 2008; **14**: 501–503.

Mendez I, Vinuela A, Astradsson A, Mukhida K, Hallett P, Robertson H, Tierney T, Holness R, Dagher A, Trojanowski JQ, Isacson O: Dopamine neurons implanted into people with Parkinson's disease survive without pathology for 14 years. *Nat Med* 2008; **14**: 507–509.

Related references

Cooper O, Astradsson A, Hallett P, Robertson H, Mendez I, Isacson O. Lack of functional relevance of isolated cell damage in transplants of Parkinson's disease patients. *J Neurol* 2009; **256** Suppl 3: 310–316.

Kordower JH, Chu Y, Hauser RA, Olanow CW, Freeman TB. Transplanted dopaminergic neurons develop PD pathologic changes: a second case report. *Mov Disord* 2008; **23**: 2303–2306.

Study design

Case studies to evaluate long-term survival and related pathology and function of transplanted foetal dopamine neurons in patients with PD.

Class of evidence	III
Randomization	None
Number of patients	7
Follow-up	Up to 16 years
	Primary outcomes: Graft survival at post-mortem Pathology at post-mortem
	Secondary outcomes: Clinical benefits Adverse events
Number of centres	3
Stratification	None

- Inclusion criteria: Idiopathic PD and pre-operative PET imaging consistent with PD. Good response to levodopa from the onset of the disease, but maximum tolerated medication not providing adequate relief of symptoms and causing unacceptable side effects.
- Exclusion criteria: Atypical parkinsonism; pronounced dementia; epilepsy; previous brain surgery; severe depression; cerebrovascular disease; and medical contraindications to surgery.

Surgical technique

- Foetal ventral midbrain tissue was collected with maternal consent from women undergoing elective abortion between 6 and 9 weeks after conception.
- Foetal ventral midbrains were dissected under sterile conditions and either single-cell suspensions or solid blocks of tissue were prepared for transplantation.
- Patients were fitted with a stereotactic head frame and the stereotactic coordinates for targets in the post-commissural putamen were calculated using MRI images and a computerized stereotactic planning workstation.
- Transplantation cannulas were inserted into the different targets in the post-commissural putamen and either a cell suspension (Li *et al.*; Mendez *et al.*) or solid graft (Kordower *et al.*) delivered along the predetermined tracts.
- Immunosuppression with cyclosporine alone (Mendez *et al.*, Kordower *et al.*) or corticosteroids, azathioprine and cyclosporine (Li *et al.*) was given post-operatively for at least 6 months.

Post-mortem analysis

- Fixed brain blocks of grafted striatum and the substantia nigra were serially cut in 40-μm thick sections on a cryostat.
- Immunohistochemistry using standard techniques was performed on free floating sections, including staining for tyrosine hydroxylase, the microglial marker, CD45, alpha-synuclein, phosphorylated alpha-synuclein, and ubiquitin.
- Immunofluorescence staining was examined using a confocal microscope and design based stereology was performed to assess cell numbers and graft volumes.

Results

Primary outcomes

- Long-term graft survival was demonstrated in all seven patients at post-mortem, ranging from 9 to 16 years after transplantation.
- Grafts contained numerous tyrosine hydroxylase (TH) positive dopamine neurons, in the order of 10,000 to 100,000 per graft.
- Grafts were well integrated and provided reinnervation of the host striatum.

- Dopamine grafts in four of the seven patients reported were found to have Lewy body-like pathology, typical of PD, as demonstrated by immunostaining with alpha-synuclein, phosphorylated alpha-synuclein, and ubiquitin. However, only an estimated 1–5% of grafted neurons in these patients contained Lewy body-like pathology, whereas the remaining grafted neurons were healthy looking.
- Solid grafts were found to elicit a stronger host immune reaction than cell suspension grafts, as demonstrated by the presence of activated microglia.

Secondary outcomes

- Clinical outcome was highly variable, ranging from little if any demonstrable benefits to marked improvements in measures of PD function, including UPDRS motor 'off' medication scores, 'off' time and dyskinesias, and substantially reduced antiparkinsonian medication requirements, with benefits lasting for over a decade. In general, the variable clinical benefits were found to correlate with the variation in graft size at post-mortem.
- No adverse events such as graft-induced dyskinesias were encountered.

Conclusions

- Transplanted foetal dopamine neurons in Parkinson's patients can survive for over a decade and provide marked and prolonged clinical benefits in a subset of patients.
- A fraction of grafted neurons can develop Lewy body-like pathology. However, this is unlikely to affect graft function.

Critique

One of the first neural transplantation studies in PD utilized dissociated foetal ventral midbrain (VM) tissue transplanted into the striatum of patients that had developed PD after accidental exposure of 1-methyl-4-phenyl-1,2,3,6-tetrahydropyridine (Widner et al., 1992). These patients exhibited marked motor improvement correlating with an increase of fluorodopa uptake in the striatum on PET scans. Furthermore, fluorodopa uptake and postsynaptic dopamine receptor occupancy PET studies have indicated that foetal grafts in the striatum can survive for up to a decade and provide sustained motor benefits in PD.

Two double-blind randomized controlled clinical trials of neural transplantation for PD in the United States have been reported. Freed et al. (2001) randomized 40 patients to receive either bilateral putaminal transplants of foetal ventral midbrain tissue from two embryos per side or sham surgery. Solid tissue was transplanted and no immunosuppression was given. The study failed to meet its primary endpoint of clinical improvement on a self-reporting scale. However, a treatment effect was observed in younger patients. Also the trial was concluded after only a year, a time that is insufficient for the growth and integration of human foetal dopamine neurons and the development of functional effects. Indeed several more patients showed clinical improvement after the conclusion of the trial, 2–3 years after transplantation surgery. Unfortunately, 'off' period dyskinesias were observed in 15% of the patients. Olanow *et al.* (2003) randomized 34 patients to receive bilateral putaminal foetal VM tissue from one or four donors per side or undergo a placebo procedure. Solid tissue pieces were transplanted. A 6-month course of immuno-suppression was given. The trial failed to meet its primary endpoint of improvement in the motor component of the UPDRS, although a treatment effect was observed in milder disease. Concerning 'off' period, dyskinesias were observed in 56% of the patients.

Few post-mortem studies of the survival of grafted cells have been reported. The studies by Li *et al.*, Kordower *et al.* and Mendez *et al.* are the first in-depth long-term post-mortem studies of the fate of grafted foetal dopamine neurons in PD. These studies have demonstrated that foetal cells can survive and integrate for over a decade in the host brain and provide long-term functional benefits. However Li *et al.* and Kordower *et al.* also demonstrated that a fraction of grafted dopamine neurons developed Lewy body-like pathology, the hallmark of PD, in their four long-term surviving patients, while Mendez *et al.* found no such pathology in their three long-term surviving patients.

To explain their findings, Li *et al.* speculated that the alpha-synuclein aggregation and deposition observed in the transplanted dopaminergic neurons was triggered by mis-folded alpha-synuclein in the host, which was transmitted into grafted cells by a 'prion-like' mechanism. Kordower *et al.* argued that abnormal Lewy body-like structures in transplanted neurons could be a result of an accelerated Parkinson's disease-like patho-logical process that affects grafted neurons possibly due to a defect in the ubiquitin proteasome pathway similar to that observed in PD. Other, perhaps more plausible explanations could be that an increased host inflammatory response contributed to the development of PD-like pathology in some of these patients or that the transplanted cells could have been affected by oxidative stress or an accelerated aging process similar to that occurring in PD.

Despite the occurrence of Lewy body-like pathology in grafted neurons of four of the seven patients reported, it should be stressed that only 1–5% of grafted neurons of these contained any pathology, whereas the vast majority of them were healthy looking. The occasional appearance of Lewy body-like pathology is therefore unlikely to affect graft function and indeed long-term benefits were observed beyond a decade in some these patients.

In conclusion, transplanted foetal dopamine neurons can survive for up to 16 years despite ongoing neurodegeneration of the host brain. Furthermore, these and several other case studies have demonstrated that grafted foetal dopamine neurons can provide substantial long-term clinical benefits in PD. These findings are encouraging for the future development of foetal and stem cell-derived therapy for PD.

Freed CR, Greene PE, Breeze RE, Tsai WY, DuMouchel W, Kao R, Dillon S, Winfield H, Culver S, Trojanowski JQ, Eidelberg D, Fahn S. Transplantation of embryonic dopamine neurons for severe Parkinson's disease. *N Engl J Med* 2001; **344**: 710–719.

Kordower JH, Chu Y, Hauser RA, Freeman TB, Olanow CW. Lewy body-like pathology in long-term embryonic nigral transplants in Parkinson's disease. *Nat Med* 2008; **14**: 504–506.

Olanow CW, Goetz CG, Kordower JH, Stoessl AJ, Sossi V, Brin MF, Shannon KM, Nauert GM, Perl DP, Godbold J, Freeman TB A double-blind controlled trial of bilateral fetal nigral transplantation in Parkinson's disease. *Ann Neurol* 2003; **54**: 403–414.

Widner H, Tetrud J, Rehncrona S, Snow B, Brundin P, Gustavii B, Bjorklund A, Lindvall O, Langston JW. Bilateral fetal mesencephalic grafting in two patients with parkinsonism induced by 1-methy-4-phenyl-1, 2, 3, 6-tetrahydropyridine (MPTP). *N Engl J med* 1992; **327**: 1556–1563.

Chapter 6

Paediatric neurosurgery

RD Johnson, P Richards, J Jayamohan, S Sinha

6.0 **Introduction**

Paediatric neurosurgery is a complex subspecialty that does not lend itself easily to large clinical trials. Outcomes may be more complex and multidimensional in paediatric neurosurgery than they are in adult neurosurgery (Kan and Kestle, 2007). In addition, there may be fewer areas where true clinical equipoise exists regarding treatment options. Nonetheless, there is likely to be an increasing number of larger clinical studies undertaken in paediatric neurosurgery over the next few years. In this chapter, four studies that highlight different aspects of the kinds of problems faced by the paediatric neurosurgical discipline have been chosen for inclusion.

Firstly, a trial of diuretic therapy for post-haemorrhagic ventricular dilatation (PHVD) in premature infants is considered (Kennedy *et al.*, 2001). This trial is important because it addresses the efficacy of a medical treatment that became widespread before any proper assessment of its clinical efficacy. The trial demonstrated that this treatment regimen may not only be ineffective but potentially increases the risk of death or disability. The second study considered is the Shunt Design Trial, which is one of very few randomized trials that examines neurosurgical devices (Drake *et al.*, 1998). The third study is a single-centre randomized trial addressing the role of decompressive craniectomy in paediatric head injury (Taylor *et al.*, 2001). Although this is only a pilot study it remains the only published randomized study to date that suggests there may be a beneficial role for decompressive craniectomy in head injury. The fourth, and final, study included in this chapter is one of the largest multi-centre trials carried out in paediatric neurosurgical patients, which examines the role of hypothermia in managing severe paediatric head injury (Hutchison *et al.*, 2008).

Drake JM, Kestle JRW, Milner R, Cinalli G, Boop F, Piatt J, Haines S, Schiff S, Cochrane DD, Steinbolc P, MacNeil N for the collaborators. Randomised trial of cerebrospinal fluid shunt valve design in pediatric hydrocephalus. *Neurosurgery* 1998; **43**: 294–303.

Hutchison JS, Ward RE, Lacroix JL, Hebert PC, Barnes MA, Bohn DJ, Dirks PB, Douchette S, Fergusson D. Gottesman R, Joffe AR, Kirkpalani HM, Meyer PG, Morris KP, Moher D, Singh RN, Skippen PW for the Hypothermia Pediatric Head Injury Trial Investigators and the Canadian Critical Care Trials Group. *N Engl J Med* 2008; **358**: 2447–2456.

Kan P, Kestle JRW. Designing randomised clinical trials in pediatric neurosurgery. *Childs Nerv Syst* 2007; **23**: 385–390.

Kennedy CR, Ayers S, Campbell MJ, Elbourne D, Hope P, Johnson A, on behalf of the International PHVD drug trial group. Randomised, controlled trial of acetazolamide and furosemide in post-haemorrhagic ventricular dilatation in infancy: follow-up at 1 year. *Paediatrics* 2001; **108**: 597–607.

Taylor A, Butt W, Rosenfeld J, Shann F, Ditchfield M, Lewis E, Klug G, Wallace D, Henning R, Tibballs J. A randomised trial of very early decompressive craniectomy in children with traumatic brain injury and sustained intracranial hypertension. *Child's Nerv Syst* 2001; **17**: 154–162.

6.1 **Diuretic therapy in post-haemorrhagic ventricular dilatation**

Details of study

This multi-centre randomized controlled trial addressed the question of whether the widespread use of drug treatment (furosemide and acetazolamide) in the treatment of PHVD in preterm infants has any effect on reducing the need for surgery by way of cerebrospinal fluid (CSF) diversion. The trial was carried out between 1992 and 1996 in 55 centres worldwide.

Study references

Main study

International PHVD drug trial group. International randomised controlled trial of acetazolamide and furosemide in posthaemorrhagic ventricular dilatation in infancy. *Lancet* 1998; **352**: 433–440.

Related references

Libenson MH, Kaye EM, Rosman NP, Gilmore HE. Acetazolamide and furosemide for posthemorrhagic hydrocephalus of the newborn. *Pediatr Neurol* 1999; **20**: 185–191.

Ventriculomegaly Trial Group. Randomised trial of early tapping in neonatal posthaemorrhagic ventricular dilatation. *Arch Dis Child* 1990; **65**: 3–10.

Study design

♦ A multi-centre PRCT

Class of evidence	I
Randomization	Drug treatment versus standard treatment
Number of patients	177 (129 with 1 year data)
Follow-up	Primary outcomes: Death or shunt placement or both at 1 year
	Secondary outcome: Neurodevelopmental status at 1 year
Number of centres	55 centres worldwide
Stratification	Presence of cerebral parenchymal lesions on ultrasonography

♦ Inclusion criteria: Age <3 months past term; ultrasound evidence of germinal or intraventricular haemorrhage; progressive ventricular dilatation with ventricular index >4 mm above 97th percentile.

♦ Drug treatment consisted of acetazolamide 100 mg/day (initiated at 25 mg/day and increased in 25 mg/day increments over 4 days) and furosemide 1 mg/day.

♦ Standard treatment included removal of CSF if head growth was double normal rate over 2 weeks or there were signs of raised intracranial pressure.

♦ Shunt insertion was recommended if: head circumference was ≥1.5 cm above 97th percentile; or head growth was ≥1.5 cm/week for 2 weeks; and presence of signs of raised intracranial pressure.

Results

◆ Follow-up was 93% at 1 year for the primary outcome.

◆ Follow-up was 83% at 1 year for the secondary outcome.

◆ Infants in the drug therapy group had a significantly increased risk ($p = 0.012$) of death, impairment or disability at 1 year. Risk ratio of 1.40 (1.12–1.76).

Primary outcomes at 1 year	Drug therapy	Standard therapy alone	Statistical significance
Death, shunt placement or both	65%	46%	$p = 0.026$

Conclusions

Drug therapy (acetazolamide and furosemide) in infants with PHVD does not reduce the rate of shunt placement and is associated with an increased risk of death, shunt placement, and neurological disability.

Critique

Post-haemorrhagic ventricular dilatation is a condition that affects 17 in 1000 infants born at less than 32 weeks gestation. With the increase in survival of neonates born at 28 weeks gestation this condition continues to be a significant source of infant morbidity and mortality.

At present the best long-term solution is insertion of a ventriculoperitoneal shunt. However, the risks of surgery and the subsequent complications of shunt surgery cannot be discounted. Several methodologies have been tried to reduce the requirement of surgical treatment, including the use of diuretics.

Diuretic drugs such as acetazolamide and furosemide can lead to a reduction in CSF production. Studies dating back to 1958 have been reported using such drugs to medically manage hydrocephalus and negate the need for shunt insertion (Birzis, 1958; Chaplin, 1980; Donat, 1980; Shinnar, 1985). Despite the lack of Level I or II evidence to show their efficacy, these drugs have found widespread usage in the treatment of hydrocephalus. Given the potential complications of diuretic therapy, the International PHVD Drug Trial Group undertook this study to address this particular issue.

The study was well designed with simple outcomes (death or shunt insertion before 1 year of age) that minimized any potential bias. In conceiving an international multi-centre trial, it was possible to recruit a large number of patients to allow a meaningful conclusion. Randomization was performed to allow a balance between the groups and within the respective participating centres.

Although it was not possible to conceal treatment allocation from the parents or doctors (in order to monitor electrolyte and acid–base status), this was not revealed to the paediatricians who carried out the neurodevelopmental assessment. It may be argued that all infants should have had their acid–base and electrolyte status assessed, which would allow blinding of the parents and treating physicians but it seems unlikely that this would have altered the outcome. Infants in either group who proceeded to shunt placement were found to have similar ventricular indices and head size, suggesting that the criteria for surgery were met equally in both groups.

The trial has been criticized for using both acetazolamide and furosemide together. However, the trial authors have argued that the risk of adverse effects from using two drugs in combination does not necessarily equate with a lack of efficacy. The mechanism of action for diuretics is the same in all types of hydrocephalus. The usage of either a single drug or differing doses is therefore unlikely to be of additional benefit. There was no evidence in the trial that any of the deaths were related to a specific biological mechanism that would implicate side effects of the diuretics. While there was an expected rise in alveolar P_{CO_2} there was no increase in the number of infants requiring ventilation.

The results show a significant increased risk of death and shunt placement as well as neurodevelopmental disability in the diuretic therapy group. There was no delay to the requirement for shunt placement with diuretic therapy. This effect was still significant after multiple logistic regression was used to negate the potential confounding effects of birth weight, gestational age at birth, post-natal age, and head circumference. The fact that the trial was stopped early due to the significant advantage of standard treatment emphasizes the deleterious effects of diuretic therapy in the treatment of PHVD.

Overall, the study was well constructed and obtained an important and significant conclusion. The authors reach a valid conclusion in stating that diuretic therapy cannot be recommended in the treatment of PHVD.

While the results of this trial were in progress, a further smaller trial was carried out at a single institute (Libenson *et al.* 1999) in which 16 patients were recruited. The results of this trial did not show a deleterious effect of diuretic therapy. However, the trial does not mention the method of randomization and there are unequal numbers in the study and control groups. Power calculations are not provided and neither the intervention nor the outcome was blinded. Subsequent meta-analysis of the two studies also reaches the conclusion that diuretic therapy cannot be recommended.

Birzis L, Carter CH, Maren TH. Effects of acetazolamide on CSF pressure and electrolytes in hydrocephalus. *Neurology* 1958; **8**: 522–528.

Chaplin ER, Goldstein GW, Myerberg DZ, Hunt JV, Tooley WH. Posthaemorrhagic hydrocephalus in the preteriminfant. *Pediatrics* 1980; **65**: 901–909.

Donat JF. Acetazolamide-induced improvement in hydrocephalus. *Arch Neurol* 1980; **37**: 376.

Libenson MH, Carter CH, Kaye EM, Rosman NP, Gilmore HE. Acetazolamide and furosemide for posthaemorrhagic hydrocephalus of the newborn. *Pediatr Neurol* 1999; **20**: 185–191.

Shinnar S, Gammon E, Bergman EW Jr, Epstein M, Freeman JM. Management of hydrocephalus in infancy: Use of acetazolamide and furosemide to avoid cerebrospinal fluid shunts. *J Pediatr* 1985; **107**: 31–37.

6.2 **Shunt design trial**

Details of study

The Shunt Design Trial assessed whether two new shunt valves could decrease the 1 year shunt failure rate compared to differential pressure valves. The study was carried out at 12 centres in North America and Europe between 1993 and 1996. The two new valves studied were the Delta valve (PS Medical-Medtronic) and the Sigma valve (NMT Cordis).

Study references

Main study

Drake JM, Kestle JRW, Milner R, Cinalli G, Boop F, Piatt J, Haines S, Schiff S, Cochrane DD, Steinbok P, MacNeil N for the collaborators. Randomised trial of cerebrospinal fluid shunt valve design in pediatric hydrocephalus. *Neurosurgery* 1998; **43**: 294–303.

Related references

Drake JM, Kestle J. Rationale and methodology of the multicenter pediatric cerebrospinal fluid shunt design trial. *Childs Nerv Syst* 1996; **12**: 434–447.

Kestle J, Drake J, Milner R, Sainte-Rose C, Cinalli G, Boop F, Piatt J, Haines S, Schiff S, Cochrane D, Steinbok P, MacNeil N for the collaborators. Long-term follow-up data from the shunt design trial. *Pediatr Neurosurg* 2000; **33**: 230–236.

Study design

Class of evidence	I
Randomization	Standard differential pressure valve versus Delta valve versus Sigma valve
Number of patients	344
Follow-up	Primary outcomes: Shunt failures at 1 year Time to shunt failure
	Secondary outcomes: Death, surgical complications Type of shunt malfunction Length of hospital stay
Number of centres	12 centres in North America and Europe
Stratification	Age (<6 months, ≥6 months) Study centre

- Inclusion criteria: Age 0–18 years; newly diagnosed hydrocephalus; radiological evidence of ventriculomegaly; requirement for first shunt insertion.
- Exclusion criteria: Previous shunt; active infection; spread of tumour to subarachnoid space; loculations requiring >1 shunt; Dandy–Walker malformation; arachnoid cyst causing hydrocephalus; systemic contraindication to shunting.

- Shunt failure defined as: obstruction; overdrainage; loculation of ventricles; infection.
- Sample size calculations were based on establishing a reduction in shunt failure rates from 40% to 20%.

Results

- Overall shunt failure at 1 year was 39% with all three valves.
- There were no significant differences in causes of shunt failure between the three valves.
- There was no significant advantage with any of the three valves.
- There were no deaths related to shunt failure.

Conclusions

There was no benefit of one valve design over another in terms of shunt failure at 1 year.

Critique

CSF shunts in the paediatric population are hampered by a shunt failure rate of approximately 40%. Shunt valve design has changed over the decades since the introduction of the first valves, but the only evidence of improved efficacy has been drawn from uncontrolled case series. The Shunt Design Trial is the first randomized trial to address the question of whether novel valve designs would have any effect on shunt failure rates.

The three valves involved in the trial were the standard differential pressure, the Orbis-Sigma and Delta valves. The latter two were designed to limit overdrainage in the upright position.

The study was well designed to attempt to answer the hypothesis. Previously published reports have shown a 40% shunt failure rate and the trial organizers felt that a reduction to 20% would show a good clinical effect. As such, the sample size was calculated to ensure the trial had sufficient power to account for such a reduction. The study was multicentric with randomization and stratified by centre and age (above and below 6 months) to optimize the trial.

The primary and secondary outcome measures used are easily defined and are non-biased. A blinded independent analysis of these outcomes was carried out, strengthening the nature of the study.

The results of the study clearly show no difference between the three shunt valve designs. The overall shunt failure rate at 1 year was 39%. Log rank analysis and Cox regression model to account for potential causes of bias failed to show any difference between the valves (log rank = 2.90, $p = 0.24$). While the sample sizes do not produce sufficient power to allow analysis for specific age groups, secondary analysis suggests that the result is valid for older children as well. The study was not sufficiently powered to assess the differences in the valve function in children with tumours in whom third ventriculostomy is the favoured option. Similarly, the nature of hydrocephalus in adults is predominantly different to that of children and it is not therefore appropriate to extrapolate these results to the adult population.

The authors rightly conclude that there is no difference between the standard differential pressure valve, the newer Orbis-Sigma, and the Delta valve in reducing the rates of shunt failure in children.

Overall the study is very well designed and represents a major landmark in being not only the first randomized trial of different shunt valve designs but also one of the very few trials of a neurosurgical device.

6.3 **Decompressive craniectomy in paediatric head injury**
Details of study

Taylor *et al.* carried out a single-centre study of early decompressive craniectomy in paediatric head-injured patients admitted to the intensive care unit at the Royal Children's Hospital, Melbourne, Australia, between 1991 and 1998.

Study references
Main study

Taylor A, Butt W, Rosenfeld J, Shann F, Ditchfield M, Lewis E, Klug G, Wallace D, Henning R, Tibballs J. A randomised trial of very early decompressive craniectomy in children with traumatic brain injury and sustained intracranial hypertension. *Child's Nerv Syst* 2001; **17**: 154–162.

Related reference

Sahuquillo J, Arikan F. Decompressive craniectomy for the treatment of refractory high intracranial pressure in traumatic brain injury. *Cochrane Database Syst Rev* 2006; **1**: CD003983.

Study design

Class of evidence	II
Randomization	Decompressive craniectomy versus medical management
Number of patients	27
Follow-up	Primary outcome: Functional outcome at 6 months
	Secondary outcome: Physiological parameters including ICP control
Number of centres	1
Stratification	Severity of brain injury

- Inclusion criteria: Age 1–16 years; severe traumatic brain injury (TBI) with functioning intraventricular catheter.

- Functional outcome was assessed using the Glasgow Outcome Score (GOS) and the Health State Utility (HSU) Index.

- Both groups received conventional medical management to control cerebral perfusion pressure (CPP) and intracranial pressure (ICP).

- Children who had uncontrolled ICP (20–24 mmHg for >30 min, 25–29 mmHg for >10 min, >30 mmHg for >1 min) were randomized.

- Those randomized to surgery underwent a bi-temporal craniotomy within 6 h of randomization.

- Favourable outcome was defined as those who were functionally normal or who had mild disability.

- Unfavourable outcome was defined as moderate disability or worse.

Results

• Follow-up was 100% at 6 months.

	Decompressive craniectomy group	Conventional medical management group	Statistical significance
Favourable outcome at 6 months	54%	14%	$p = 0.046$ ($p < 0.0221$ required)
Mean reduction in ICP post-randomization	8.98 mmHg	3.69 mmHg	$p = 0.057$

• There was a non-significant trend towards a shorter time in intensive care in the decompressive craniectomy group.

Conclusions

There may be an advantage in early decompressive craniectomy in the paediatric patients with severe traumatic head injury in terms of control of ICP and favourable outcomes. However, a larger multi-centre trial is required to assess this further.

Critique

Decompressive craniectomy remains a rather controversial area. There is often a strength of opinion among clinicians either for or against it without any significant evidence to back either view. To date, there is no Level I or II evidence in the adult population that addresses this issue. Two studies are in progress (RescueICP and DECRA) that hope to provide evidence in the near future for the adult population. Given this background, the study by Taylor *et al.* tries to address this aspect in the paediatric population.

The study was well performed with attempts to remove any bias. It struggled, however, in a number of ways. The study took 7 years to perform and despite this only 27 patients were recruited. The authors mention that clinical management policies changed during this period but one would expect that these changes would affect both arms in a similar fashion.

Patients were selected if they had a traumatic brain injury and had a functioning intra-ventricular catheter. Diffuse brain injury often leads to cerebral swelling without increase of ventricular size and often significant compression of the ventricular system, contraindicating the placement of such a catheter. The majority of patients with diffuse injury are usually managed with an intracranial pressure monitor and may not have been included in this study.

The surgical treatment can also expect some criticism. Craniectomy was performed by removal of 3- to 4-cm discs of bone bi-temporally with no attempt to open the dura. Studies looking at expansion have showed that a large craniectomy with dural opening is required in order to maximize the benefit of craniectomy. Perhaps with a more definitive decompression more significant results may have been seen.

The outcome analysis was described as being carried out by telephone interview, chart review, and/or discussion with the treating physician. While the unit has significant experience of follow-up in this fashion, outcome measures are more accurately achieved by both clinical and neuropsychological review. Functional outcome measures in children were carried out at 6 months only with no further evaluation. It has been shown that outcome status in children changes over time and it would have been useful to have reassessed outcome at 1, 2, and 5 years to give a more long-term picture.

Due to the changes in management protocol over the study period, statistical analysis was performed on two separate occasions. The results showed a favourable outcome in 54% of patients in the decompressive group compared with 14% in the control (medical) group. Using the two-tailed Fisher's test, $p = 0.046$, but owing to the repeated analysis the p value for statistical significance is reduced further to $p < 0.0221$, leading to the conclusion that early decompressive craniectomy may have a beneficial effect.

Despite some of the above-mentioned shortcomings, the study by Taylor *et al.* was well designed and performed. The results, while not statistically significant, do suggest that there is likely to be a benefit from early decompressive surgery. Given the difficulty of recruitment in a single centre and the limitations of studies with small numbers, the authors rightly conclude that a larger multi-centre trail is required to further address this important question.

6.4 **Hypothermia in paediatric head injury**

Details of study

The efficacy of hypothermia in the management of paediatric head injury was examined in a multi-centre international trial by the Hypothermia Paediatric Head Injury Trial Investigators and the Canadian Critical Care Trials Group between 1999 and 2004 in North America.

Study references

Main study

Hutchison JS, Ward RE, Lacroix JL, Hebert PC, Barnes MA, Bohn DJ, Dirks PB, Douchette S, Fergusson D. Gottesman R, Joffe AR, Kirkpalani HM, Meyer PG, Morris KP, Moher D, Singh RN, Skippen PW for the Hypothermia Pediatric Head Injury Trial Investigators and the Canadian Critical Care Trials Group. *N Engl J Med* 2008; **358**: 2447–2456.

Related reference

Clifton GL, Miller ER, Choi SC, Levin HS, McCauley S, Smith K, Muizelaar JP, Wagner FC, Marion DW, Luerssen TG, Chestnut RM, Schwartz M. Lack of effect of induction of hypothermia after acute brain injury. *N Engl J Med* 2001; **344**: 556–563.

Study design

Class of evidence	I
Randomization	Hypothermia versus normothermia
Number of patients	225
Follow-up	Primary outcomes: Morbidity and mortality at 6 months
	Secondary outcomes: Overall mortality Co-intervention requirements Physiological variables Functional psychological outcomes Adverse events
Number of centres	17 centres in three countries
Stratification	Age < 7 and ≥7

- Inclusion criteria: Age 1–17 years; GCS <8; CT evidence of brain injury; need for ventilation.

- Exclusion criteria: >8 h post-injury; brain death; cervical cord injury; prolonged cardiac arrest; non-accidental injury.

- Patients in the hypothermia group were cooled to 32.5°C within 8 h of injury and therapy was continued for 24 h.

- Patients in the normothermia group were kept at 37°C.

- Paediatric cerebral performance category scale (PCPC) was used to assess outcome. This is a 6-point scale: (1) normal performance; (2) mild disability; (3) moderate disability; (4) severe disability; (5) persistent vegetative state; (6) death.
- Unfavourable outcome was defined as a PCPC score of ≥4.
- Favourable outcome was defined as a PCPC score of ≤3.
- Analysis was performed on an intention-to-treat basis.

Results

- Follow-up was 91% for primary outcome data.

	Hypothermia	Normothermia	Statistical significance
Unfavourable outcome at 6 months	31%	22%	$p = 0.14$
Overall mortality	21%	12%	$p = 0.06$

- The degree of hypotension and requirement for vasoactive agents in the hypothermia group during the re-warming period was significantly greater than in the normothermia group.
- Significantly more interventions were required to control ICP in the normothermia group within the first 24 h compared to the hypothermia group.

Conclusions

Hypothermia initiated within 8 h from injury and continued for 24 h is not associated with improved neurological outcome and may increase mortality in the paediatric population.

Critique

While animal models suggest that hypothermia improves survival in traumatic brain injury the evidence for a similar response in children has remained lacking. Hutchinson *et al.* therefore designed this trial in order to explore the outcome following hypothermia therapy after traumatic brain injury.

This was a prospective multi-centre randomized study encompassing 17 centres in three countries. The study was well designed with a simple primary outcome, which was assessed by persons blinded to the original assigned arm of treatment. A secondary outcome to assess neuropsychological changes was carried out by telephone by a trained psychologist, as well as interviews with parents at several time-points following injury.

In order to reduce any potential bias, the management protocol for both arms was decided by consensus prior to the study, allowing for comparison across all the centres. Randomization and stratification was carried out according to each centre and by age (grouped into <7 or ≥7 years). The latter was fashioned as children sustaining significant injuries at a younger age have poorer neuropsychological recovery than older children. The criteria for cooling were based on best-published evidence at the time of the trial.

Statistical analysis incorporated adequate power calculations and took into account potential losses to follow-up. An interim analysis at two separate points was used to ensure that the trial should not be stopped. Results were analysed on an intention-to-treat basis and logistic regression used to account for factors that could adversely influence the results.

The follow-up at 6 months was 91%, which was in keeping with the predicted power calculations. There was no significant benefit from the use of hypothermia when the primary and secondary outcomes were analysed.

Sensitivity analysis used to account for the patients lost to follow-up when biased against hypothermic treatment suggest a significant risk of an unfavourable outcome in the hypothermia group ($p = 0.001$). However, when biased towards normothermic treatment, the results showed no increased risk in the hypothermia group ($p = 0.82$).

Subgroup analysis for primary outcome showed no significant difference between the two treatment arms except in patients in whom the ICP remained less than 20 mmHg. In this particular subgroup, hypothermia treatment had an increased risk of an unfavourable outcome (RR 2.12, $p = 0.03$).

In a subgroup analysis of secondary outcome, there was a significant trend to poorer visual memory in the hypothermia group when assessed at 12 months ($p = 0.05$).

The mean time taken to achieve hypothermia in these patients was approximately 6 h. It may be argued that perhaps earlier institution of cooling may have a better outcome as is seen in animal models (15 min to cooling), however, the practicalities of assessment and treatment in children with severe head injury make faster treatment highly unlikely. The authors mention that unpublished results looking at a subgroup of children who were able to be treated early showed no benefit either.

Hypothermic treatment was only used for 24 h in this study, which may not be long enough to optimize its beneficial aspects. There is some evidence that treatment for more than 48 h may reduce the risk of death and an unfavourable outcome in adults (systematic review—McIntyre et al., 2003).

Although the study ran over 5 years, the numbers of children recruited was only 225. Small treatment effects are unlikely to be detectable with such a small sample and leaves room for a larger trial to explore other potential benefits.

While there are some aspects that could be improved upon, the trial was well designed. The two treatment arms were well matched for management with no significant co-interventions that would bias the results. It would be of benefit to reassess the children at further intervals, as outcome status in children changes over time. This would provide a more long-term picture.

A more recent systematic review and meta-analysis by the Cochrane Collaboration in 2004, showed no overall benefit from either immediate or deferred hypothermia treatment in adults with severe brain injury. This meta-analysis included the McIntyre review (mentioned above) in which the suggested beneficial results were obtained by pooling results from both deferred and immediate hypothermia studies.

The outcome of the trial reaches a valid conclusion that hypothermia for 24 h is not beneficial in the management of severe head injury in children but still leaves questions about potential benefit of earlier or a more prolonged treatment in certain subgroups of patients. Further larger trials would be required to assess these more specific aspects.

Alderson P, Gadkray C, Signorini DF. Therapeutic hypothermia for head injury. *Cochrane Database Syst Rev* 2004; **4**: CD001048.

McIntyre LA, Fergusson DA, Hébert PC, Moher D, Hutchison JS. Prolonged therapeutic hypothermia after traumatic brain injury in adults: a systematic review. *JAMA* 2003; **289**: 2992–2999.

Index